DENTAL
SCHOOL
INTERVIEW

Questions and answers with full explanations

2nd edition

Sri Hari Ravi MBBS Bsc (Hons)
Veena Babu MBBS Bsc (Hons)
Risha Patel BDS

Simon Cowen Publishing

SIMON COWEN PUBLISHING

Ordering Information:
Quantity sales. Special discounts are available on quantity purchases by corporations, associations, and others. For details, contact the publisher at the address above.

Orders by UK trade bookstores and wholesalers.
Please contact Medinterview;
Or visit www.medinterview.com
Printed in the United Kingdom.
All content is owned by the authors.

Publisher's Cataloging-in-Publication data
Copyright © 2015 by Simon Cowen Publishing

1st Edition 2013
2nd Edition 2015

ISBN-13: 978-0990853800

ISBN-10: 0990853802

CONTENTS

INTRODUCTION

Applying to dental school can be a daunting experience, to say the least. But it needn't be. This book provides the ultimate resource for prospective students looking to overcome that last hurdle- the Dental School Interview!

Having helped hundreds of students ace their medicine and dentistry interviews, the authors have meticulously put together this resource with their top 'know-hows' on common pitfalls alongside the 'Do's' and 'Don'ts' for the most commonly asked questions.

We recommend using this book as a preparatory tool alongside other appropriate reading materials. Traditional UK Dental School interviews have been one to one (with the interviewer and student) or panel based (with a panel of interviewers and the student). More recently however, these are being replaced by MMI (multiple mini interviews) styled interviews. The latter is gaining popularity as an objective overall assessment tool, that helps to gauge the candidate's caliber by getting them to problem solve on the spot. Here, the student moves from one interviewer to the next in the form of timed 'stations' focusing on different aspects of the interview. The first step is knowing what type of interview you are preparing for; make sure to ring the university to double check so that there are no surprises on the day.

Needless to say, first impressions, intertwined with your ability to formulate articulate answers on the spot are what will win over the interviewing panel. So how do you do it? The answer is simple. Practice. Practice. Practice. The more you practice, the less nervous you will be and your answers will sound a lot more confident. Use the sample questions in this book to practice with others or in front of a mirror, in order to build upon your confidence and style of delivery.

The twelve easy to digest chapters have been devised in an insightful way using a combination of tips, explanations and model answers for you to work from. We recommend using the model answers as a framework to formulating your own examples to the questions, particularly in respect to attributes that will make a good dentist. For instance, it would be beneficial to think of some personal examples where you have demonstrated skills such as leadership, communication, team work , manual dexterity, empathy, decision making etc.

We advice that alongside this book you keep up to date with current dentistry news within the NHS, the media and your local dentist.

Purchase of this book gives you a £50 discount on the day interview course which is run by the authors of this book. The course includes full teaching and preparation for the interview and a mock MMI circuit.

Please enter code – VBitloml397 when purchasing the course at medinterview.com.

Chapter 1

GENERAL POINTS TO CONSIDER

You are understandably feeling a concoction of emotions at present, comprised of ingredients such as anxiety, uncertainty, excitement and surmounting pressure. We want to assure you that with the right guidance, preparation and practice you can and will succeed in your dental school interview. Not letting the pressure get to you is pivotal in determining your overall performance, and as you work through the chapters in this book, we hope that you build upon your knowledge and confidence, alike. This chapter will home in on some general points to consider when preparing. We suggest that you keep referring back to this chapter throughout, so that you don't forget the key basics.

Your answers

We strongly advice that you prepare answers for the most commonly asked questions by learning them in bullet points. This will ensure that you articulate the answer differently each time and will   save you from appearing over-rehearsed. Give natural responses and expect the unexpected in regards to questions you will be asked, as failure to do so can make you come across as inflexible.

Use ethical terms appropriately when answering questions, the genuine consensus amongst interviewers is that inappropriate use of terminology often makes the candidate seem like they are trying too hard to be something they are not (in this case intelligent). Therefore, do not be too polished in your answer, be as natural as possible, the interview process will give you ample opportunity to highlight your strengths.

Maturity can be demonstrated when you reflect on a question asked by including your personal experience and achievements (make sure it is genuine, as being caught out on a lie will not be taken lightly by your interviewer). You need to help paint a picture in the interviewer's mind about your experiences, in order to demonstrate your passion and credibility.

Example:

Have you ever worked in a team?

" Yes, I have worked in a team on several occasions both academic and socially. For instance, I was part of a Elderly Outreach team from my sixth form and I thoroughly enjoyed working alongside my peers. On the other hand, I regularly play football and hockey

and have to exercise good listening and team work skills in order to ensure the best for our team"

In regard to specific questions asked:

Try and answer all questions in detail; see the bigger picture and give your answers putting the question into context taking into account all situations/circumstances, examples of how to do this are given consistently throughout the book.

Try and emphasise your appreciation of complex questions, however when presenting your answers be clear and concise.

The use of good English is vitally important so take your time when answering questions, you are not expected to roll answers of your tongue, nonetheless, you are expected to consider questions carefully before answering. Do not fall into the trap of answering questions instantaneously, you will be more likely to make a mistake with your grammar and once again it will not seem natural. Some examples of colloquial/slang words to avoid:

"cool"

"yeah"

"things like that"

When describing your personal qualities demonstrate an even balance of confidence, intelligence and humility. Do not sound too brash, only use your achievements as illustrative examples when answering questions, remember the interviewers have your personal statement; you have already impressed them enough to have gotten this interview. Always provide examples when answering questions about you, do not just talk in theory.

Be prepared for your personal statement to be scrutinized (particularly common in a panel/traditional styled interview). Alongside your personal qualities, be prepared to demonstrate skills of manual dexterity. Interviewers appreciate you bringing examples along(miniature models that you have made, pictures of cake decorating, knitting etc), however, this might not be feasible for the MMI. Ring the university beforehand to check whether you should bring examples/pictures or any models.

When answering questions regarding why you want to be a dentist- be honest and demonstrate a realistic understanding of a dentist's roles and responsibilities. The General Dental Council (GDC) recognise 13 dental specialties that you should be familiar with. Furthermore, you could then elaborate on any key interests e.g. paediatric dentistry, periodontics etc. Demonstrate your caring ability, but also give clear reasons why you want to be a dentist compared to other healthcare professions such as a doctor.

Key points to consider

The detailed role and routine of a modern day dentist.

Examples of how you have prepared for the interview.

Examples of how you have developed the qualities to be a dentist.

Demonstrate enthusiasm and passion for the vocation show that you want to find out more about a career in dentistry.

Remember there is no model answers for the question "why do you want to be a dentist?" The answer to this is unique to you as an individual but must contain some shred of wanting to be intellectually challenged alongside enjoying the personal relationship that you get to share with your patients.

Demonstrate a realistic perception that you know why dentistry is the only career for you. While doing so, ensure that you don't belittle other careers such as medicine or nursing, but instead compare them to the role of a dentist and justify why the former is more suited for you.

Body Language

Your body language represents a key part of the screening process for dental school. After viewing your personal statement and assessing your predicted grades, most universities will call those they are seriously considering of offering a place to an interview and this will be your final opportunity to show them why you are deserving of studying Dentistry.

Body language incorporates many features. It includes the way you dress, act and react to questions during the interviewing process. Therefore, it is imperative that this section goes into detail on what is required of you when this time comes as it could be the difference on just missing out or being offered a place at Dental School.

Do's + Don'ts

By studying Dentistry you will be required to meet members of the public on a daily basis. The public want to be cared for by someone who they hold in high esteem and can be looked upon as a respected individual. Therefore they will judge you even before you start to speak to them. One must therefore strike an image of the characteristics above by displaying them to the interviewer so he/she can be assured you meet the credentials of a future doctor.

**Shaking the interviewer(s) hand before you begin may highlight your professional manner and is advisable, but not necessary.

Body Posture

At all times keep your back straight and avoid slouching when walking and sitting down. If you are someone who fidgets or are restless, place both your hands together and place them on your lap. However, do not shy away from using your hands during dialogue-but do not over do this as it can become very distracting for the interviewer! As a woman, crossing your legs when wearing a skirt should be done to avoid embarrassment. Men should also attempt to cross their legs but keeping their legs moderately together is equally acceptable.

Getting someone to film you while you practice is a great way of seeing how you come across in an interview. You can then alter your posture/body language appropriately.

Gestures + Facial Expressions

By all means feel free to express yourself as this often emphasises how well you can communicate your feelings to others- a good characteristic when working in a team. React well to jokes and good news with smiling and laughter but show concern and sadness when presented with less favourable information. In essence, the aim is to convey that you can communicate in a manner appropriate for a situation (this should be no different to how you would react when talking to a friend!). It is highly advisable to be clean shaven before the interview and to make sure your hair is neatly cut and not interfering with your face.

Eye Movements

This is vital when in conversation with the interviewer. Maintaining eye contact shows that you can engage well when in conversation and are not easily distracted, it shows the interviewer that you are a confident individual and, most importantly, makes the interviewer feel a lot better about talking and listening to you. This feature of body language should not be downplayed as it can easily lead to a poor interview if not executed well. If you are in a panel interview and have more than one person questioning you, maintain eye contact with the person questioning you and do look/smile at the others in the room from time to time. If the interviewer does not smile back or respond to your gestures , do not be disheartened and don't let this throw you off. They are trying to be objective and won't want to appear over friendly, but this is by no means an indication of how you are doing in the interview.

Clothing

For the interview we advise that men should wear a 2 piece suit with a tie and polished shoes. The colour should not be too bright, ideally black, navy blue or grey. Women have slightly more freedom in that they have a choice of a skirt or trousers with a blouse/shirt. A matching jacket can also be worn. We advice that you check your tops by leaning forward/bending to ensure that they are appropriate and not too revelaving; this is to be fully prepared in case a station requires you to actively do a task, whereby you will be confortable in your attire. Women should also wear polished shoes but avoid high heels. Remember to dress with an aim to look smart and professional.

Do not feel afraid to showcase any badges from college/high school which show off your current achievements (e.g. Prefect/ Head Boy badges), but keep this to a minimal. We advice that you keep makeup, cologne/perfume, hair products etc tᴗ minimum. There should be nothing about your demeanour that distracts the interviewer from your answers.

Before you move on to the next chapters we want you to start structuring your thoughts and thereby your answers to common questions. This will make your answers concise and articulate. The following framework is recommended.

POINT

Answer the question with your point

EVIDENCE

Build on the answer with a personal life example/experience.

EXPLANATION

Link this to the future, either as a prospective dental student, as an individual or a citizen of society etc

ample:

ʊ

ι you deal with pressure?

- " *I believe that I can deal with pressure as I have been under pressure on several occasions. Most recently, I had to represent my school at an inter-school talent competition and found that talking to family and close friends helped me lighten my stress load. I look forward to all the future situations that I will face under pressure as I know that it will aid my growth as an individual.*"

We cannot emphasize the importance of having a good structure to your answers and would strongly advice that you pick a framework best suited to you and apply it to your answers as you work through the questions in this book.

RESOURCES

http://www.bdasmile.org – To understand things/cases from a patient's perspective

http://www.dentalhealth.org/- Regular updates on news and articles in the dentistry world

http://www.bmj.com/search/dentists - Read a few papers weekly,to widen your knowledge

http://www.nhs.uk/NHSEngland/Healthcosts/Pages /Dentalcosts.aspx- Read about dental costs and how it affects the NHS

http://www.medicalnewstoday.com/releases/252954. php- Some more articles to give you a wider understnading

The website of the university that you will be attending for the interview- it is crucial that you browse through these, paying close attention to the following:

Research carried out at the university

Their societies and student groups- particularly any that you would like to join and contribute to

Details specific to their programme

15

<u>Notes</u>

Chapter 2

TRADITIONAL INTERVIEWS AND MMIS (Multiple Mini Interviews)

Part of being well prepared, is the art of knowing how to prepare. This will rely heavily upon the interview style that you will be subjected to. This chapter is designed to give you an insight into the two most common interview styles that you will come across.

We advise that you double check with your respective universities about their style of interviews; you can also easily access this information on their official website. This chapter will hopefully highlight to you the importance of not being put off by anything unexpected during your interview (whichever style)- the more you learn to relax the better your performance will be.

The dental school interview itself can be one of two styles:

Traditional – an interview with one or more academics on a panel in a formal or semi-formal setting. These can last anywhere from 20 minutes to an hour. The candidate remains in the same room for the entire period of the interview.

MMIs- a series of short, structured interview stations lasting approximately 7 minutes per station and consisting of around 6-10 stations. Here the candidate, moves from one station to the next after the given time frame. Each station may have one interviewer or an interviewer and a designated actor.

Traditional Interviews

What are traditional Interviews?

This style of interviewing has been in place for many years; it consists of a short interview with an interviewer or panel of academics. This is usually a dentist, doctor, an admissions tutor, or a senior member of staff at the institution. The purpose of this interview is to familiarize themselves with the candidate beyond their personal statement and grades.

Likewise, you must ensure that everything you have stated in your personal statement is credible, otherwise you will get caught out and that could be the end of your application process. The interviewers are interested in gauging your personality, critical reasoning skills, communication skills and your ability to deal with given problems.

In the interview itself, do not be put off if only one member of the panel speaks to you and the other/s are taking notes, this may simply be for administration purposes and shouldn't worry you. However, ensure that you greet every individual when you enter and leave the room for courtesy. Similarly, don't get thrown off course if the interviewer reacts to something you said in an unexpected way. Instead, take a second to gather your thoughts and carry on.

What will the interview comprise of?

This type of interview will involve a mixture of questions similar to the topics covered in this book. However, these questions won't necessarily be divided in to subtopics. The interviewers may go back and forth between topics depending on the tone of the interview. You could also be given problems to solve on the spot, either abstract, ethical or quantitative and will be assessed on how you work under pressure.

How should I prepare?

Candidates in the past have found it useful to treat the interview as a performance, whereby, they remind themselves not to get too comfortable at any point. Keeping this in mind will warrant that you keep everything from your body language to your answers to a good standard. Use the interview process to build rapport with your interviewer. Let them see who you are, don't be afraid to smile or even laugh when appropriate. Don't let the nerves of the situation transform you into a robot with mechanical answers.

When preparing for this style of interview, practice with a group of friends/family members and get feedback on your body language, posture and all the other aspects of non-verbal communication from Chapter 1. You can then aim to improve your performance with each practice run, based on your feedback.

MMIs (Multiple Mini Interviews)

This is a newer method of interviewing candidates which has recently found favour by many medical and dental schools alike. Once again, there should be nothing that throws you off course if you have a rough idea of what to expect from these mini interviews.

What are MMIs?

For dental schools, there are typically 6- 8 stations (varies from school to school), each lasting around 6-10 minutes. The candidate should enter each station with a brief introduction and answer the respective questions in that station before thanking the interviewer and moving on to the next station. All the stations will be right next to each other and the interviewer stays put while the candidate moves from one desk to the next.

What will the stations comprise of?

The principle challenge here is that candidates need to repeatedly make a good first impression and build rapport whilst performing well. The stations will be divided into topics almost like the chapters in this book. For example, you may have one station where you will discuss your work experience and hobbies, whereas another may involve you discussing the challenges of being a dentist for the NHS. Therefore, it is vital that you answer questions in a concise and articulate fashion.

In the ethical scenario station, you may be given a case to read and then discuss with the interviewer. Read it carefully, and think of all the issues that come up which you should bring to focus. Don't rush in to deliver your answer, but instead gather your thoughts and quickly plan which side, if any, you will take or how you will critically analyse the given case study.

Some universities have an abstract station where you may be presented with a picture or an object and asked to simply elaborate on what you see. This is not to throw you of course. The interviewer wants to see how well you can relay information, a skill considered vital for dentists. If presented with an image, we suggest that you state what you see on a whole and then home in on details of the picture.

Remember to think about the attributes that make a good dentist and using examples try to frequently demonstrate to the interviewer, how you possess these attributes.

Some examples of stations from the last four years :

- Ethical scenario debate
- Quantitative task (calculator provided)
- Physical task testing manual dexterity. some examples include:
a. Making a paper aeroplane using instructions

b. Making a paper boat using instructions

c. Doing tasks on the ipad

d. Abstract station – candidates are required to interpret a given image

- Personal qualities and "why this university?" styled questions
- "Why dentistry over other careers?" styled questions

Universities using MMI's for admission in 2015:

Aberdeen
Birmingham
Bristol
Cardiff
Dundee
Glasgow
King's
Leeds
Liverpool
Manchester
Plymouth
Queen's Belfast
Queen Mary
University of Central Lancashire

Tips on dealing with actors

There will usually be at least one station with an actor. The scenario will always be within your limits. For example, your vignette may read:

Your neighbour, Mrs X is just coming home. Please speak to her about her window- which you accidentally broke while playing cricket with your friends

You are a volunteer at a dental practice , please speak to this patient who has been waiting for over an hour to see the dentist and is quite cross

You are a volunteer at a shelter, please help this blind man cross the room by verbally giving him instructions

Irrespective of your given scenario, remember to always start with an introduction,

For example:

"Good afternoon, my name is Peter Richards and I'm one of the volunteers here, would it be alright if I assisted you today? May I please get your name..."

Always be honest and sincere and be creative in trying to find solutions to help them. This is where most of your marks will lie. Be apologetic if the actor is getting anxious/agitated, and offer practical solutions such as a glass of water, some magazines while they wait etc.

Thank the actor and examiner at the end of the station before moving on. You may find that you have completed the station with ample time to spare; don't be alarmed- this is quite common. Keep in mind that in the remaining time if something comes to mind that you would like to add, you still can.

How should I Prepare?

Time management is key to performing well in the MMIs. Eight minutes will go quite quick and you want to make the most of each station. For instance, make sure you don't waste time thinking about the perfect example where you demonstrated leadership skills, but instead, have these pre thought and ready to use.

Similarly, do not panic if you are faced with a problem that you cannot see the solution to straight away. It may help to think out aloud as the interviewer will gain insight in to your thinking process- which is always better than two minutes of silence. In case you get cut off mid-sentence and the bell goes off to move to the next station, don't forget to thank your interviewer before moving on or else you can wave goodbye to the rapport that you spent the last eight minutes building. Even if for some reason you slip up in a station and don't do as well as you thought, try and get it out of your mind before you move to the next station. The last thing you want is a negative domino effect on your performance in the other stations.

For your preparation, get into groups with your friends and set up mock stations to practice with-you'll be surprised how useful this turns out to be in the run up to your interview. Practicing like this is the best way to build up your confidence and better your time management skills. Keep a journal with their feedback and use it to improve your performance to the most commonly asked questions, using examples from this book.

Chapter 3

SCIENCE BASED QUESTIONS

Remember that dentistry is a science and although you won't be expected to know some of these answers, it will aid your thinking process and provide a good foundation for other answers.

- Describe how cancer is formed?
- How can we reduce risk of a heart attack?
- What are the causes of smoking?
- What have you read recently about genetics?
- Do you think bowel cancer is common in the UK?
- What can be done to help ovarian cancer?
- How does MRI work?
- How does Ultrasound work?
- What is the structure of DNA?
- What is Down's syndrome?

The key to answering a science related question well is to take what may be a complex topic and to present it clearly and simply. If you do not know the answer it is okay to let the panel know this information; however, by going through the questions in this chapter you should get a rough idea of how to tackle a majority of topics. We advise you to go away and read around any topics which come up here, which you are unfamiliar with.

'Patient.co.uk' is a brilliant resource for answering science questions in a clear way without using jargon (dental terms). It's sometimes helpful to give a brief definition/overview of the condition as an introduction. If unsure, do not try and bluff your way through an answer as the examiner will see through this. As mentioned before, prior to answering any question, take a minute to gather your thoughts and formulate an answer.

What do you understand about how cancer is formed?

Cancer occurs when previously normal cells become abnormal and multiply uncontrollably at a faster rate than normal. This can lead to a cluster of abnormal cells called a tumor. The cancer can be classified as malignant, which is when the tumor has invaded surrounding organs, or benign which does not invade other organs.

How can we reduce the risk of heart attack?

A heart attack is when part of the heart muscle dies, due to a clot preventing blood flow to the heart itself. This deprives it of oxygen and thus the heart cannot then pump appropriately, leading to a reduction in the amount of blood passing round the body. It is known that some people have a higher predisposition to getting a heart attack based on their family history, which makes it all the more important to take active measures to reduce your risk. The risk of a heart attack can be reduced by making a few lifestyle changes, Some of which include:

Healthier diet: more fruits and vegetables, low fat, eating foods containing 'good' cholesterol

Stopping smoking

Taking up exercise- 5 sessions of 30 minutes each week. Vigorous enough to make you slightly out of breath.

3. How does smoking increase your risk of cancer and cardiovascular disease

Cigarettes contain cancer causing agents known as carcinogens, which can cause mutations in cells. When cigarettes are smoked, carcinogens are released into the body, and can eventually lead to cancer. The longer a person smokes the more carcinogens they are exposed to; and therefore, the higher the risk of cancer, especially lung and mouth cancer.

Smoking also causes narrowing of blood vessels, which increases the risk of an individual suffering a stroke or heart attack. The more a person smokes, the narrower their vessels may become, therefore, increasing their risk of cardiovascular disease

4. What have you read recently about the role of genetics in science

In answering questions about research try and find a broad topic rather than a very niche topic. It is more relevant that you are aware of main issues at the moment, and it's more likely you will be able to answer questions on a broader topic.

For Example:

"There has been a lot of work on looking at the effects of genetics on ageing, and scientists are trying to determine if particular genetic make-up makes you more susceptible to degenerative diseases such as Alzheimer's. Researchers at Kings College London have discovered biomarkers for Alzheimer's disease. I find all this very fascinating and cannot wait to explore the topic further when at university."

5. Do you think bowel cancer is common in the UK, explain your answer? (this is just to get you thinking and is highly unlikely to be asked at a dental school admissions interview)

Even if you do not know how common bowel cancer is (3rd commonest cancer in the UK after lung and breast) you can use the answer to this question is to demonstrate your knowledge of current medical issues, as over the last few years bowel cancer screening in older individuals has increased in importance, highlighting that bowel cancer is an issue.

For Example:

"I think that bowel cancer is a common issue in the UK, based on medical literature (e.g. the BMJ and other medical journals). There has been a drive towards promoting bowel cancer screening, particularly in those over 65, as this leads to early diagnosis. In turn, this enables people to receive necessary treatment earlier, increasing the chances of complete recovery. I love how science is constantly changing and adapting to meet the emerging needs of the public. It is interesting to note how research heavily influences any change in policy/ screening measures and I personally think this is an area where more resources(e.g. money) should be invested by the NHS."

6. What can be done to help prevent cervical cancer?

This question is testing your knowledge of public health campaigns, in this case the HPV (human papilloma virus) vaccine and cervical smear testing.

For Example:

"Cervical cancer is one of the commonest cancers occurring in women, but unfortunately is often detected too late for treatment to be effective so there are campaigns to help prevent cervical cancer. The first is by the HPV vaccine which is given to girls of a secondary school age to prevent the spread of viruses which are known to increase the risk of cervical cancer. The second is by cervical screening, where the cells of a woman's cervix are examined once every few years to look for changes to cell structure, as that can sometimes be an indication of cancer."

7. How does MRI (magnetic resonance imaging) work?

MRI is a method of scanning the body using radio waves and a large magnet; therefore, without the risk of radiation. The patient lies down a couch and is passed through the MRI scanner, which resembles a short tunnel. As the patient passes through the scanner, the radio waves and the magnetic field formed by the magnet create a detailed picture of all the organs and bones, as well as any foreign bodies such as tumours.

'Patient.co.uk' is an excellent resource for most if not all types of medical investigations. It is definitely worth reading through some of the more commonly performed investigations such as ECG, X-ray, MRI, Ultrasound etc.

8. How does an Ultrasound machine work?

Ultrasound is a painless way of viewing organs and structures inside the body using sound waves, which are transmitted through a hand held probe. Cold lubricating jelly is put on the skin to be scanned, and then the probe is held to the skin. Ultrasound waves are then sent through the probes. As the ultrasound waves hit the bones and organs and bounce back towards the probe, a picture of all visible internal structures is formed.

9. What is the structure of DNA?

It sounds simple but answer the question, you are being asked about the structure of DNA, not about DNA in general. Try to explain this question simply, without using lots of jargon as that could confuse you (unless you know the topic well).

For Example:

"DNA, or deoxyribonucleic acid is made up of a number of different molecules. The backbone is two strands of nucleotides, which run in opposite direction, and therefore are antiparallel. Nucleotides are made up of a base, a sugar group and a phosphate group. There are four bases, adenine, thymine, guanine and cytosine. As they all have unique structures, adenine is always joined to thymine on the opposite strand, and cytosine is always joined to guanine. The strands are joined by ester bonds. The bases occur in a specific sequence, determining the genetic code."

10. What do you know about Down's syndrome?

Down's syndrome is one of the commonest types of genetic disease. It occurs when a person has three copies of chromosome 21 instead of two, usually due to a genetic mutation. The older the mother, the higher the risk of her baby having Down's syndrome. This is particularly significant in women over the age of 40. The risk of Down's syndrome can be assessed during pregnancy, and if a mother is found to be at high risk, a mother can be offered amniocentesis, a test which can determine if a baby has Down's syndrome. However, this test carries a high risk of miscarriage. Down's syndrome is associated with a number of other medical condition, most common being problems with the structure of the heart.

Chapter 4

ETHICAL BASED QUESTIONS

Ethical dilemmas can present themselves to you at anytime and in any environment. They are not restricted to your career after graduation, they can often occur during Dental School itself. Due to the nature and responsibility of a dental professional to their patient, team and the public, most universities like to see the student's reaction and thought process when faced with such situations.

The 'General Dental Council (GDC)' (Standards for Dental Professionals, May 2005) outlines the following as principles and responsibilities in the practice of dentistry:

- Putting patients' interests first and acting to protect them.
- Respecting patients' dignity and choices.
- Protecting the confidentiality of patients' information.
- Co-operating with other members of the dental team and other health care colleagues in the interests of patients.
- Maintaining your professional knowledge and competence.
- Being trustworthy.

When faced with an ethical scenario it is useful to bear these principles in mind in order to give an appropriate and balanced answer. At home, try to brainstorm other responsibilities or qualities you think it is important for a dentist to have and later in the chapter see which questions you may be able to apply these to when answering.

Ethical scenarios won't always be in the context of a dentist. You could also be given scenarios which are closer to home whereby, you need to apply the ethical principles and give a balanced answer. Some examples include:

You see your friend has cheated in an exam- what do you do next and why?

 you see your sibling stealing from a shop- what do you do next and why?

 you notice your colleague stealing money from the register – what do you do next and why?

<u>Answering Ethical Questions</u>

When answering ethical questions, there is usually no single right answer. This is important to understand as most candidates waste precious time thinking about the "perfect answer to give". The aim of many of these questions is to be able to consider the situation from many different perspectives. Ideally you want to:

Identify all relevant themes and issues

Present a balanced argument

In some cases you may wish to:

Culminate with your opinion and a definitive answer IF the question requires it.

However, it is important to be careful that you do not allow your opinion to dominate your answer and prevent you from showing that you have considered all options.

The four pillars of ethics include Autonomy, Beneficence, Non-Maleficence and Justice. Other important ethical areas concern confidentiality, capacity, competence and consent. These are common themes that are repeatedly raised in dental school interviews, therefore invest some time familiarizing yourself with these terms and their application.

All of these are explored and explained through the practice answers below.

You can use the practice questions below to apply the above. If you are struggling to give a balanced argument practice by creating a table of 'pros' and 'cons' in your head with a minimum of three points in each. Alternatively, you can consider structuring your thoughts via each person in the situation and what their roles, opinions and potential problems may be.

Example Ethical Questions

- If I gave you £100,000 to go to countries in the developing world, how would you use it?
- If, on a scale of 0 to 5, 0 was caring for people and 5 was an interest in science, where would you put yourself on the scale?
- One day, a colleague gives you a sheet containing questions for an upcoming exam. How would you handle the situation? What issues would you consider important in coming to a decision about what to do?
- How do you handle the situation where one of your patients does not speak English? What issues can you see potentially arising in this situation?
- Patient Confidentiality is of utmost importance in a clinical profession such as dentistry. Are there any circumstances where the disclosure of patient information may be justified?
- Do you know the four ethical principles of medicine?
- Do you think there is a role for individuals with physical disabilities in dentistry?
- Is it fair for the NHS to spend time and resources on patients who have self-inflicted diseases/problems?
- Is it right for dentists to have personal feelings for their patients?

- Do you think dentists should have the right to ever strike?
- What do you know about the General Dental Council?
- Consider the case of nine year old Rebecca who comes in to your surgery with her parents. This is her first dental visit. She has been kept awake with a painful tooth.
- Examination shows that she has several decayed teeth and that a lower right primary molar is causing the present pain.
- Rebecca is crying and climbing out of the dental chair. What is the best way to handle this situation?
- Why do you think the suicide rate in dentists is so high?
- What are the arguments for and against banning selling tobacco?
- What is more important; quality of life or length of life?
- Do you feel that you would feel emotion if a patient died during an incident in your surgery?
- What do you think of stem cell research and the possibility of using it to treat diabetes?
- Would you empathise or sympathise?
- Do you believe an alcoholic has the same rights as a non-alcoholic to receive treatment and transplants?
- Do you believe euthanasia is acceptable, explain why?

If I gave you £100,000 to go to countries in the developing world, how would you use it?

It is easy in an interview where your end goal is attaining a place in dental school to jump straight into the nitty gritty of solving all the dental problems in the world. Take a step back and think of the big picture before homing in on the specifics. Try to think of sensible (not necessarily medical) ways of spending money which would address issues in the developing world. For example, donating money towards:

Water sanitation to ensure constant clean water supply to tackle conditions such as gastroenteritis in infants.

Academic resources such as exercise books, textbooks and writing tools in underprivileged communities and schools

In these countries, sustainable projects which have a long lasting impact on the community are also a brilliant way to help. Consider:

The buying and growing of crops and farm equipment in rural areas to form a sustainable food supply/provision of long lasting edible goods. In the interest of a balanced argument you can also consider raising a point about possibility of goods falling into the wrong hands and ending up on the black market.

If you would like to include a dentally related answer it is important to remember that in developing countries their dental needs vary dramatically from those you see within the UK. Focus your answer on projects such as:

Raising awareness for both children and adults about preventative measures which should be applied on a regular basis. Consider the area you may wish to target and whether to take aids with you. These could include toothbrushes, toothpaste, models to demonstrate oral hygiene instruction and positive reinforcement for children such as stickers. Sticking to the idea of creating a long-term impact, you could also consider a further training programme for adults within the community allowing them to be able to deliver your oral hygiene education to other members of the community and within schools to more children.

Raising awareness for projects focused on detecting and preventing oral cancer. The World Health Organisation (WHO) found that oral cancer is the second most common cause of death in developing countries causing 7.1million deaths in 2003 with an estimated 50% rise in the number of new cases over the next 20 years. Education for people in these countries is paramount and money can be wisely spent saving lives.

(The World Health Report 2004: changing history. The World Health Organization and International Union

If, on a scale of 0 to 5, 0 was caring for people and 5 was an interest in science, where would you put yourself on the scale?

As dentistry combines the compassion to care for people as well as an interest in science, it wouldn't be advisable to select either 0 or 5 as that would imply you lack one of the core attributes of being a dentist.

If you answer within the middle of the scale give a balanced argument for both points. If you decide to place yourself towards either end of the scale make sure you not only illustrate why you have done so and why one attribute weighs more heavily in your individual favor but also acknowledge the other quality as being important in dentistry.

You can consider giving examples of areas where you have already shown commitment and talent to these attributes.

For example:

"As I have a strong interest in both caring for people [highlighted through my work experience at...] and an interest in science [which I furthered during my project on...], I would put myself as a 3. I think it is essential to have a good balance in these interests as I feel both of these attributes are essential for a dentist to be successful and responsible."

day, a colleague gives you a sheet
taining questions for an upcoming exam.
..v would you handle the situation? What
issues would you consider important in
coming to a decision about what to do?

This questions your knowledge of ethics and your
ethical backbone. They want to know that you would
do the right thing if faced with this scenario.
Remember whilst this scenario may be more likely to
present to you at school or college, they are testing
how you will be in the future; as a dentist in practice.
In practice, a scenario such as this may have
implications for patients, who may be at risk or the
law may have potential to be broken. Remember the
principles of dentistry discussed at the beginning of
this chapter. The GDC expect you to 'put patients'
interests first and act to protect them' and 'be
trustworthy'. The GDC further encourage 'whistle
blowing' in cases where patients are at risk or the law
is broken. Therefore, as a professional you cannot sit
back and let this scenario happen.

Take your time discussing all the issues raised. These
include:

Trust in your colleague

Whether you colleague has any serious problems
going on affecting their ability to learn or revise the
syllabus

Whether your colleague actually understands and

remembers the content and the potential future risk of not knowing the content

Mention the pillar of ethics that relate to the scenario, in this case- Justice

For example:

"In this instance I would first want to know where the questions came from, how they were acquired and why my colleague felt he/she needed to use them. Cheating the system is very dangerous and has very serious implications when you get caught; I would make my colleague aware of this and would not partake in cheating. I pride myself in working for the results I achieve and cheating would not validate them at all. I would discourage them from using this sheet and advise them to either, give the sheet back to where they got it from, or hand it in to staff. If they adamantly refuse having known the implications and consequences of what they are doing I would have to warn them that I would report them if they did not take steps to amend the situation. If no action was taken by them I would report this case to the relevant members of staff, detailing any further concerns I may have had from our initial conversation."

o you handle the situation where one of patients does not speak English? What can you see potentially arising in this situation?

This situation highlights this principle set out by the GDC; 'Respecting patients' dignity and choices'. Here, consent for examination and treatment will be a key issue. In order for consent to be valid, it must be:

Voluntary: the decision to consent or not consent to treatment must be made alone, and must not be due to pressure by medical staff, friends or family.

Verbal- for example, when the patient directly gives permission

Implied- for example, when a patient rolls up their sleeve for a blood pressure reading

Written- for example, in cases where the patient may need to go under general anaesthetic for an operative procedure

Informed: the person must be given full information about what the treatment involves, including the benefits and risks, whether there are reasonable alternative treatments, and what will happen if treatment does not go ahead. Healthcare professionals should not withhold information just because it may upset or unnerve the person.

Capacity: the person must be capable of giving consent, which means they understand the information given to them and they can use it to make an informed decision.

(NHS Choices 2012)

You can see that with a language barrier it is not possible for consent to be valid. It would also be difficult for the dentists to fully understand what the patient has come in for and potentially lead to an incorrect diagnosis and treatment.

In this situation you can ask if any other members of staff speak the language and can aid in translation. If not, you can ask if the patient can bring in a translator before any treatment is carried out. You must make sure the translator fully understands what you are saying and relays the information accurately and without embellishment or coercion to make consent voluntary. To avoid this problem you can use a translation service that will provide you with a qualified translator for the appointment. There are also leaflets and pictures available detailing common treatments in various languages which can be used an aid but not on their own to gain consent.

Patient Confidentiality is of utmost importance in a clinical profession such as dentistry. Are there any circumstances where the disclosure of patient information may be justified?

It is important to remember that all personal information belongs to the patient, not to the dentist. Therefore in any circumstance whereby the patient has permitted disclosure of any personal information to a third party most commonly; other healthcare professionals participating in the care of the patient, insurance companies seeking information or solicitors acting for the patient, the disclosure is justified. It is often prudent to gain both verbal and written consent for this. *Showing Care*

However, in cases where disclosure without the patient's consent or even their knowledge occurs you are at risk of disregarding the GDC principle of 'protecting patient confidentiality'. It is extremely rare for dental records to be called upon whereby the patient cannot know or give consent, but they do exist. It is acceptable to disclose information without consent only if it is in the public or individuals interest. For example; with regard to the individual's health and safety being put at serious risk or help preventing or detecting a serious crime. In these cases always be prepared to justify your decision.

"Even though the clinician has to respect patient confidentiality at all times, there may be some situations where this may be over looked; if it in the public or individual interest. For instance, in legal requirements, in case of certain infectious diseases (NOT HIV), serious injury or dangerous situations or when ordered to do so by court possibly in identification of missing or deceased persons. During my work experience placement I learnt from the dentist that often the only way to identify human

remains will be dental records. This in ι
relieve the distress of relatives involved, heι
criminal cases and thus be justifiable."

Another key fact to remember with regarc ιo
confidentiality and information that is not relevant to
this question but can come up is not only are you
responsible for not disclosing information, you must
also ensure no one has <u>unauthorized access</u> to any
information. This does not confine itself to written
records alone, it includes speaking about patient's in
open environments where this information can be
overheard and used by a third party.

Do you know the four ethical principles of medicine?

1. Respect for Autonomy - the patient has the right to
refuse or choose their treatment

2. Principle of Beneficence - a practitioner should
always act in the best interest of the patient

3. Principle of Non-maleficence – a practitioner
should never do harm to a patient

4. Principle of Justice – this is about the distribution
of scarce health resources, and the decision of who
gets what treatment

you think there is a role for individuals with physical disabilities in dentistry?

The answer here is never 'no'. There should be no discrimination due to disability in any field of employment. A model answer would be:

"If an individual's disability does not reduce their capacity to learn and action what is required to practice dentistry, care for their patients and impart knowledge to others, then yes I feel there is a role for these individuals in healthcare. However, I feel it would need to be acknowledged that such individuals may have specific needs that need to be addressed. These could include methods to help them learn more effectively, appropriate and comfortable environments to take exams etc"

Is it fair for the NHS to spend time and resources on patients who have self-inflicted diseases/problems?

This question is a good example of a case where your personal opinion may dominate the answer, preventing you from giving the well-balanced reply that is desired.

A background of the NHS will help to answer this question. The NHS was set up with the aim to provide quality care to everyone. In 2011 the NHS Constitution outlined seven key principles regarding treatment and service patients could expect. Principle One highlighted the need for equality of care regardless of gender, race, religion, marital status etc and this includes the individuals personal involvement in causing their condition. Principle Four further stated that the NHS 'should support individuals to promote and manage their own health'. So if they are to blame, as clinical professionals we have a duty to educate them on any measures they can take from this point on.

For Example:

"As the NHS was created to provide quality care to everyone, even if their condition is self-inflicted, our job is to treat these individuals. But, in this current economic climate and the financial problems the NHS are facing, we cannot ignore the time and resources lost treating these individuals, which could have been used on other patients. This places an emphasis on the need for further education. Rather than lay blame on these patients, I think it is more important to take preventative steps which would reduce the number of individuals with self-inflicted diseases; promoting healthy lifestyles such as reducing alcohol intake, stopping smoking and encouraging a healthy diet and exercise."

Is it right for dentists to have personal feelings for their patients?

I do not think they are interpreting personal feelings here as romantic feelings. It is understood that you know romantic feelings let alone actions are unacceptable so unless you want to find yourself pulled up in front of the GDC before you even become a dentist do not say you think romantic feelings are allowed!

A well balanced and concise response would include:

"As dentists are first and foremost people, it is normal that some patients may evoke feelings of frustration, joy, sadness or even anger. However, it is important that dentists are able to prevent these feelings from clouding their judgment both positively (being more attentive to one patient at the detriment of the other) and negatively (as a prejudice of a prior belief)."

Do you think dentists should have the right to ever strike?

The key here is remembering as dentists you always put the patient first. See the answer below for the degree of balance required when answering:

"A dentist's first responsibility is towards their patients and their care. Any action which would compromise this would be questionable. However, the world is not black and white and dentists are individuals who also have the right to earn a living in

a job they are comfortable and happy in within reasonable parameters. So if they decided they needed to take a stand against something, and all other appropriate action had been attempted before a strike considered, I think there may be circumstances whereby dentists are allowed to strike, providing they ensure patient care is not compromised."

What do you know about the General Dental Council? GDC

This council was established in 1956, by a Dentists Act, thereby creating an independent profession. Until then, the General Medical Council held overall responsibility for dentistry, although some business was under the responsibility of the 'Dental Board of the UK'.

The GDC is the self-regulatory governing body in Dentistry. It aims to protect patients and instill faith in the dental profession. It does this by regulating dentists, setting and maintaining standards and improving quality of care where necessary. They deal with those working outside of the law to the detriment of the patient.

You will unlikely need to know any details regarding the GDC but will need to understand their role in affecting patient care. If you would like any further information their website which is accessible to everyone will have everything you need.

Consider the case of nine year old Rebecca who comes in to surgery with her parents. This is her first dental visit. She has been kept awake with a painful tooth.

Examination shows that she has several decayed teeth and that a lower right primary molar is causing the present pain.

Rebecca is crying and climbing out of the dental chair. What is the best way to handle this situation?

Clinically Rebecca's case draws on various themes. Without starting your undergraduate training you will not need to know about the clinical implications in detail. However, an understanding of the themes will make you stand out. A common answer is to indicate that some dentists may consider writing a brief referral letter to the local hospital for this tooth to be extracted with a general anaesthetic. The questions that you want to be thinking about clinically are:

Can this tooth be restored or does it need extraction?

What are the implications if I extract in the future (orthodontically can it have consequences)

Does the patient need General Anaesthetic or can this be managed within practice under Local Anaesthetic.

Rebecca has other dental needs as stated and has never attended a dentists before, how would I like to manage this to cause her the least upset?

All of the above would require consideration of who would be consenting for the patient. In this case at 9 years old, the patient would require a parent or legal guardian to consent for her.

'Gillick Competence' allows for a child up to the age of eighteen to make their own decision regarding their care. However, the dentist must carefully assess that all the criteria for valid consent detailed in question four are present. There is particular emphasis placed on the patient's ability to understand and retain all the information given and communicate their reasoned decision. 'Gillick Competence' will be more relevant for scenarios where the child in question is slightly older.

The ethical and legal responsibility to respect children as well as those who support them is essential in establishing strong professional relationships. In this particular situation explaining the options and offering choices will help the parents to make their decisions appropriately after understanding what's on offer, which in turn will increase the likelihood of co-operation, whichever option is finally decided upon.

For Example:

"The dentist should tell the family about the options and explain how the pain can be controlled with

analgesics and a simple dressing. He /she should explain that it may be wise to slowly introduce Rebecca to dental care so that she becomes familiar with the dental environment before starting treatment. In this way he is enforcing the act of beneficence by acting in the patient's best interests and enabling the child's parents to make an informed decision- thereby enabling autonomy"

Why do you think the suicide rate in dentists is so high?

Dentists often undergo severe mental and psychological stress due to the nature of their working life. They will see patients from many different backgrounds, with different behaviors and attitudes. Their days will often be very busy, changing regularly as and when emergency patients need to be seen, with pressure to meet individual or practice targets whilst maintaining the high quality care all patients deserve. Outside of their jobs they also need to find a way to balance their professional lives with their personal lives where they may also be experiencing difficulties.

Often clinicians feel they cannot talk to others about their problems, as it was previously seen as a sign of weakness to show that one needed help, which lead to dentists internalizing their problems. In some cases dentists simply feel lonely as they work in small practices where there aren't many people to talk to if they so wish.

Unfortunately, in quite a number of cases, the problems experienced are serious enough that dentists feel they cannot cope and feel there is no way out other than suicide.

Furthermore, dentists often have access to potentially life-threatening medications alongside the knowledge with which to use them to cause harm, and as such any attempted suicide is more likely to be successful.

However, with more information and personal experience dentists are now increasing the forums they have to speak about their worries and problems, or merely socialize if that is what they need. Attitudes towards needing to use these types of peer groups have become much more positive giving many more dentists the chance they need to realize they are not alone in the daily problems they face.

What are the arguments for and against banning selling tobacco?

These types of questions are asked to see whether you are able to think laterally about a controversial topic. It is important to look at both sides of the question as it specifically says "for and against".

There are many ways to tackle this question and it is a

good one to practice making a mental 'pros' and 'cons' list in your head with three items in each column.

For Example:

"With the occurrence of lung and oral cancer constantly on the rise, tobacco selling is still a controversial issue. Tobacco selling should be banned as the accessibility leads to an increase in the number of younger people who take up smoking, education on its effect is present but not everyone has easy access to the full details and the effects of passive smoking can be fatal. This can be particularly unfair in cases involving younger children who cannot leave a room their family member is smoking in or do not understand the potential consequences of being in the room to make the decision to leave.

However, as all individuals have the right to choose whether to smoke or not, putting a blanket ban on the sale of tobacco may lead to the recurring argument that Britain is turning into a 'nanny state'. With all GPs and Dentists and many nurses and clinical professionals trained in smoking cessation advice it is also becoming much easier for patients to access a form of support when they do wish to stop themselves so an argument can be made to focus on education."

What is more important; quality of life or length of life?

Quality of life is an important factor in medicine and dentistry in determining the impact of disease, medication, or any intervention on a person's life. It is usually regarded as more important than the length of a person's life in medicine.

For Example:

"Although we would all like to live long lives, above all I believe it's more important to live a fulfilled life, no matter its length. Therefore I think quality of life is more important than length of life."

To think outside of the box on this question however, let's consider how often a treatment option or consequence in dentistry will commonly cause death. There are not many, excluding cases of oral cancer. So if we are considering dentistry alone we can think that life refers to the lifespan of the tooth and so the length it can be retained in the mouth can sometimes trump the quality of the work to be done.

For example, consider a child that has a deciduous (baby) tooth which has a cavity and questionable prognosis, with the treatment options being to extract and remove the possibility of infection or pain from the tooth or to remove the decay and place a temporary dressing until it is ready to naturally come out to preserve space for the permanent (adult) tooth. The second option may be preferred because even though quality may be sacrificed as pain and infection may ensue; in the long-term keeping the tooth for as long as possible may prevent orthodontic work.

Do you feel that you would feel emotion if a patient died during an incident in your surgery?

A question like this is trying to ascertain whether you understand the range of emotions you will feel in case of a complication or unexpected situation, while recognizing the emotional strength that is needed to be a good dentist. A similar question testing the same thing could include a scenario where you have a child being abused.

For Example:

"Being human, I think I would feel emotion if a patient died, such as sadness for the patient and their family, anger that despite our best efforts a patient still died, or even relief that the patient's suffering has ended.

I know that in dentistry there will be lots of scenarios which cause me to feel emotion including the discovery or suspicion of an abusive relationship, a disagreement with a team member or a difficult patient. But I appreciate that this accompanies the nature of the job and need to find a healthy way to deal with those emotions and conduct myself in a professional manner".

What do you think of stem cell research and the possibility of using it to treat diabetes?

Whilst this question is not fundamentally related to dentistry it can come up as a way to test your knowledge of current affairs especially in the field you wish to embark your further education in. Where possible try and think outside the box of any links to a topic within dentistry that you can incorporate into your answer.

For Example:

"Stem cell research has been an exciting area of medicine over the last few years, as it was suggested that stem cells could be used to regenerate organs. Although progress has been made it seems it would be still years before stem cell research is used widely to cure what are known as autoimmune diseases (diseases where the body does not recognize a particular organ as being a part of itself and it

begins to attack it, e.g. diabetes (where the pancreas is affected) and thyroid disease. In diabetes it is thought stem cell research could be used to 'grow' another pancreas using the patients' own stem cells, and see whether this would stop the body attacking it.

At present, scientists at the Dental Institute at King's College London have been successful in using stem cells to grow new teeth in mice. Human trials are still on hold but this is a massive move forward in the field of dental research and sounds very promising for the future."

Would you empathize or sympathize?

The definition of empathy) is the ability to identify with another person's feelings and emotionally put oneself in the place of another. Sympathy is feeling pity or sorrow for the misfortune of others.

For Example:

"Even though sympathy is our normal reaction to hearing someone's bad news, I would empathize more than sympathize as I think it is more important for a patient to know that their doctor/dentist knows how to understand what they are going through; even without going through it themselves; then have

a doctor/dentist who just feels sorry for them but cannot relate to the situation and use this to put them at ease."

Do you believe an alcoholic has the same rights as a non-alcoholic to receive treatment and transplants?

Another medically related question, but here the focus of your answer lies in not being judgmental.

For Example:

"As one of the foundations of medicine is that everyone has the right to receive treatment without prejudice, regardless of their lifestyle, I believe alcoholics have the right to receive treatment. However, as a prerequisite for receiving a transplant, evidence that the patient will look after the transplanted organ is needed. In the same way a smoker would be required to give up smoking before receiving a transplant, an alcoholic is not eligible to undergo a liver transplant unless they show evidence that they have stopped drinking. As long as the patient has stopped drinking for the required amount of time, the patient is entitled to receive a transplant in the same way as any other patient."

Do you believe euthanasia is acceptable, explain why?

Another good example of the interviewers desire to see balance in your answer, without too much focus on your topic in relation to dentistry.

For Example:

"I believe in cases where a patient has a disabling illness which decreases their quality of life substantially, and where the chances of recovery are slim to none, I believe euthanasia may be acceptable only if suggested by the patient themselves. As doctors are primarily promoters of health I do not think it is appropriate for doctors to ever suggest this. Nor is it acceptable for them to make the decision on the patient's behalf.

However, I do not think euthanasia is an acceptable option for every person suffering from a chronic illness, as many people with chronic illnesses are still able to maintain a good quality of life. To define which cases are acceptable and which aren't could prove difficult as each individual case will vary and people experience of their quality of life is subjective to their own past experience, opinion and expectations."

64

Notes

Chapter 5

ABOUT THE UNIVERSITY

1. What do you know about the way we teach dentistry?

2. What do you know about the intercalated BSc?

3. What extra-curricular activities would you consider joining here if you were offered a place?

4. What will you bring to this institution, not mentioning your academic achievements?

5. What are the qualities about our dental school that least attracts you?

6. What do you know about PBL (problem based learning)? Why do you want to come to a PBL based dental school?

7. Why do you want to attend our dental school?

8. How are you a match for our dental school?

9. How do you study? How does that correlate with our dental school?

10. What do you look for in a good dental school?

1. What do you know about the way we teach dentistry?

Research the course at each university you are applying to as there are significant differences between them. This information can easily be accessed via the university website or course prospectus. Know whether your course is traditional (i.e. 1 year of lecture based medical sciences followed by 4 years of clinical sciences), integrated (where you learn clinical science alongside medical science and e-learning), problem based learning (where teaching is based around a problem presented. This type often includes a lot of self-study) and whether the course includes dissection of cadavers, or whether simulated dissection takes place.

For Example:

"At X univeristy, the dental course is taught quite traditionally. During the first two years teaching is very lecture based, mainly focusing on the medical sciences such as anatomy, biochemistry and physiology, as well as including basic clinical skills in treating minor gum problems and starting to provide dental care to patients. During the 'clinical' years, teaching is less structured, and more learning is attained on the clinics. However occasional lectures still occur."

2. What do you know about the intercalated BSc?

For Example:

"The intercalated BSc is a one year degree programme which can be obtained alongside your dental degree. It can be taken after the second, third or fourth year of the dentistry programme. Although this degree is usually in a medically related subject, such as Pharmacology or Physiology, there is wide variety of programmes available, which vary by university. The intercalated BSc provides a student with the opportunity to study an area of interest in detail, with the potential to undertake research and have that research published. You thereby graduate with a BDS Bsc."

3. What extra-curricular activities would you consider joining here if you were offered a place?

This question is a chance to 'show off' your previous sporting or artistic achievements, or to show an aspect of your personality by talking about different activities you would like to be a part of.

You may choose to go onto University's student union website, have a look at what clubs and societies are held, and decide which activities you would be interested in. If you choose a slightly unusual group/society be prepared to discuss why.

For Example:

"Having played netball to a high standard at my school, I would relish the opportunity to represent my university in this way. Furthermore, I would also be interested in joining the volunteer groups X and Y; which both involve working with children from surrounding areas and deprived schools; as I was involved in mentoring younger students at school, and found it humbling to see the positive impact on the children involved."

4. What will you bring to this institution , not mentioning your academic achievements?

Similar to the question above, this is an opportunity to talk about your previous non-academic achievements in the context of activities that you would like to continue, or you can go onto the University's student union website and decide which activities appeal to you.

For Example:

"Being a keen singer, I would like to join the university choir. Further, having played football during my scholastic years , I look forward to freshers' trials to get the opportunity to represent my university in inter-university games. Additionally, as I have been involved in charity work during school, I would like to continue this in some form at university.

As I am also interested in doing volunteer projects abroad I would like to combine the charity work and volunteer projects I would be interested in groups such as Tenteleni or the Kenyan Orphan Project."

5. What are the qualities about our dental school that least attracts you?

When asked to comment on a negative aspect of something always say how you could/would overcome it, as this will demonstrate your ability to overcome obstacles in your future.

For Example:

"As X School of Dentistry is the largest dental school in the UK; its least attractive quality may be the size of the cohort. Although it would be amazing to study here, if I was fortunate enough to gain a place at this dental school, I would ensure I knew who to contact if I required any academic or personal support."

6. What do you know about PBL (problem based learning) ? Why do you want to come to a PBL based dental school?

PBL (problem based learning) is something all prospective dental students need to be aware of, even more so if you are applying to a University that teaches by PBL, such as the university of Manchester etc.

PBL is a relatively new way of facilitating learning amongst dental students. Opposed to the more traditional way of teaching (known as didactic) by lectures, PBL presents students with a 'problem' in a tutorial, and with the help of a facilitator they address the issues raised in the problem and work together towards the solution.

For Example:

"I would like to go to a PBL type dental school as I feel that I learn better by being more actively involved in my teaching, by being able to have discussions with peers, as opposed to being sat in a lecture room with 100 other students. I also think that if I had to actively seek the answers to particular problems, I'd remember them better which in turn will aid my learning in the long run. "

7.Why do you want to attend our dental school?

Show them you have done your research on the university that you are applying for. Is it the university's accolades? Is it the course structure? Is it the demographic of people you will treat? Is it the clubs and societies you want to join/create? Did your work experience dentist attend that university?

You need to find some things that make the university

different to other universities, as well as thing they pride themselves in and why you like things/how they relate to you.

"I want to come to your university because having done some reading on the course structure I really like the early exposure to patients and the way the course progresses from theory to practical work. I enjoy working with my hands so the sooner the better! The culture and diversity in London means I am sure to see a lot of variation in patients with conditions I may not see elsewhere but in London. This university has great history and it is known that the student who graduate from here are taught very well, I would like to be one of them, I am ready to work harder than before to become everything this university wants me to become."

you a match for our dental school?

on from the previous question in that you
w that you have done your background
he university and are aware of things you
do (other than study) at the university.
Check out the universities SU (student union) website
to look up clubs and societies, so that you are aware of
a couple of things that you would like to try out.

For Example:

"This university prides itself in graduating very talented dentists, I feel that I have the creativity, passion and want to be one of these graduates and this university has the resources I would like to get me there. I would also like to come and join the basketball team here as they are quite successful and sport is something I thoroughly enjoy as a break from work. I also hear there are a number of charity shows and performances organised by students for students and this is something I would love to be a part of. London is a very busy city which reflects myself very well, I am a person who likes to be kept busy and occupied with something, if you want anything done give it to a busy person."

9. How do you study? How does that correlate with our dental school?

This is just reflective of you as a person. University gives a lot more freedom to students to study in their own time and your interviewers need to know that they can trust you to put in the hours when not in lectures or in clinics to ensure that you keep on top of your work for your exams. DO NOT SAY 'I'M A LAST MINUTE CRAMMER'!! A question like this requires you to demonstrate you time management, organization and planning skills.

For Example:

"I work steadily throughout the year, studying further into things I either don't understand or find interesting. I enjoy learning as it's not a chore. So often I find myself learning more than was 'necessary' for topics. King's is renowned for it's research which is a lot of work of individuals/teams back. This is something I am used to already and would love to bring this hard-working mentality to Kings."

10. What do you look for in a good dental school?

Again this will exhibit you as a person and what you are looking for from dental school. A good social life is not a bad thing but this should not be top of your list. Try to match what you look for to what the course offers, to further cement the reason you want to be at this university.

For Example:

"I look for a university with excellent teaching and learning facilities, this has those. I also look for a place that gives good student satisfaction (which I have read this university recently does- look at the recent Times league tables to see where the university placed for student satisfaction etc). I can work well in large or small groups (I think I will do very well in this university because of that). I look for a school with enough good dental facilities to teach their students well, and I look for good access to staff as ad when needed. These are all things this university has which is why I have applied here."

Chapter 6

PERSONAL QUALITIES ABOUT YOU BASED QUESTIONS

Questions:

1. What qualities do you possess which will help make you a good dentist one day?

2. What qualities make a poor dentist?

3. Why not medicine or nursing as a career?

4. How has your academic journey been thus far?

5. Do you know of anyone in the dental/medical profession, if so have they influenced you in any way to become a dentist?

6. What do you do to relax?

7. Sell yourself to us for 2 minutes?

8. What are the most important attributes for maintaining good working relationship between colleagues?

9. Do you read, what was the last book you read?

at genre of films or books are you most
ted in?

e you a people person or do you prefer to
be alone?

12. Do you enjoy working in a team?

13. Have you ever experienced death?

14. How do you deal with stress, as dentistry is
a very long and stressful subject to study?

15. Tell me about any of the situations where
you have shown leadership skills.

16. In ten years time after you have become a
doctor and all your friends want to have a
reunion but you are unable to attend, how
would you want them to remember you?

17. How can you relate being a doctor to
playing competitive sport?

18. Have you ever considered taking a gap
year?

19. What did you do for Duke of Edinburgh?

20. Have you ever had to make an unpopular
decision as a leader?

21. Do you believe your communication and
organisational skills are adequate to become a
great dentist?

22. What would you describe as your worst qualities?

22. What would you describe as your worst qualities?

23. How would your closest friends describe you?

24. How do you handle criticism?

25. Give me an example when you have had your opinions overridden, what did you do?

26. What person(s) has had the biggest positive impact on you?

27. How have you developed your communication skills?

28.Give examples of you showing that you have good dexterity?

NOTES

1. What qualities do you possess which will help make you a good dentist one day?

To answer this question, you need to know the qualities encompassed by most good dentists. Most dental schools have a list of qualities they expect dentists, and therefore dental students to have.

This can usually be found on their website or in the prospectus so it is worth having a look through that list. When answering personality-based questions such as this, rather than just listing qualities, pick two or three and provide evidence that you possess these skills.

For Example:

"The aspect of putting my love for science into clinical practice, where I can constantly interact with an array of patients using manual skills and a sharp perceptual ability is what draws me to dentistry. I have always paid meticulous attention to detail in school projects and my extracurricular activities and I believe this quality will pay off when I gain more clinical exposure to various dental scenarios.

I am certain that my passion for people and for science entwined with my good communication skills, provide a good foundation, which if built upon appropriately would make me a good dentist."

2. What qualities make a poor dentist?

Begin by saying how although individuality among dentists is encouraged, there are certain qualities which would not be helpful within the dental field.

Such qualities include

- Poor timekeeping
- Inability to work in a team
- Poor communication skills
- Poor record keeping
- Poor manual dexterity

3. Why not medicine or nursing as a career?

Remember here that you are to exhibit some knowledge about how dentistry differs to other health care professions. So don't just say you'd prefer a '9-5 job' or that the salary is attractive! An excellent way to demonstrate this would be using examples from your work experience with a dentist and that with a doctor/nurse/ on a ward and comparing the difference between each patient –clinician interaction.

"I am passionate about people and being a dentist will enable me to put my clinical knowledge in to

practice and build a unique relationship with patients as I will see them regularly and not only when they are ill. Furthermore, the facet of treating patients manually really appeals to me. I want to build rapport with my patients and take them through the whole process, from diagnosing their condition, investigating it and treating it. Arguably GP's have a similar role as they do this for a number of common conditions, but they need to refer to a specialist for a wide variety of cases too."

4. How has your academic journey been thus far?

This is a straightforward question and the answer here will be personal to you. Try and highlight relevant areas of your academic journey to keep the answer focussed yet relevant.

"As with most journeys, my education has been generally smooth. Some parts have been very rewarding, such as winning academic prizes during my time in school and sixth form, and other parts have been somewhat more challenging, but I have managed to overcome them. I know that if given the opportunity to begin a degree in dentistry, that there will be greater academic challenges ahead, but I will try and find methods to overcome them."

5. Do you know of anyone in the dental/medical profession, if so have they influenced you in any way to become a dentist?

The following model question is for people who have dental professionals in their social/family network. However, if you have no family or friends in the dental profession you can discuss how a family member's encounter with dentists has influenced your decision to be one. On the other hand, the simple fact that you don't personally know anyone within these professions could be enough drive for you to want to enter it yourself.

"My aunt is a dentist, and hearing the passion she had for her job, made me want to find out more about the profession. Furthermore, on doing some work experience with her at her clinic, I admired the way she interacted with patients and always tried to do her best for them.

It showed me how important good communication skills are in dentistry, as they can determine whether or not a patient follows your advice. Due to her influence I have tried to improve my communication skills as well as maintain a good level of academic achievement."

6. What do you do to relax?

This question is just to show the panel that you know how to relax, and have a life outside of dentistry. It does not need to be anything over the top, rather something realistic and unique to you.

"I like to relax at home with family and friends watching films or just catching up. I also like to play netball and play the piano to relax. I ensure that I make time to do things that relax me as it enables me to work more effectively."

7. Sell yourself to us for 2 minutes?

With questions such as these it is important that you say things about yourself that you can back up if possible, e.g. by talking about achievements, prizes, anything that makes you stand out.

"Not only am I academically able, as shown by the prize I won at school for academic excellence and all round achievement, I also have a wide range of interests. I have played cricket for my school, including representing the school at the National Independent Schools Tournament, winning both a gold and silver medal in the competition.

I am also quite musical, having played the piano for

a number of years, and achieving a grade 5 in piano. I also sing in my church, and have sung with the Royal School of Church Music on a number of occasions. I love working with children, and have done so over the last 2 summers as a nursery nurse assistant."

8. What are the most important attributes for maintaining good working relationship between colleagues?

Good working relationships are important to improve the flow of information, develop an understanding of each other's views, reduce tensions and disagreements, and also to improve efficiency within any working environment.

This is even more pertinent in the multidisciplinary team setting within the practice of dentistry today.

"Good communication is essential to any team environment, to make sure everyone knows what's going on, and to ensure that the team are all working toward the same goal. This will further promote a culture of honesty and transparency which will only strengthen patient-dentist relations and enable dentists to provide more efficient overall care as a result."

9. Do you read, what was the last book you read?

This question will help the interviewer to gauge your interests further.

"I love to read, the last book I read was called 'Handle with Care' by Jodi Picoult. This is about a child born with severe osteogenesis imperfecta whose mother takes the decision to sue the doctor who delivered her child for wrongful birth. The book details how each member of her family handled the illness, and the impact of the trial on each on them. I found this book exhilarating and found it really difficult to put down"

10. What genre of films or books are you most interested in?

This question again is to gauge your non-academic interests.

"I enjoy a wide variety of books and films, but mostly drama and comedy. I love watching a plot unveil itself and particularly enjoy watching movies where I have read the book beforehand. It is always interesting to see how the film maker's interpretation of the book differs from my own imagination of the set and its characters, from having read the book ."

11. Are you a people person or do you prefer to be alone?

"Generally I am a people person, and enjoy activities like going out for meals with friends, but from time to time I enjoy being in my own company as it helps me gather my thoughts and reflect on recent events and plan future projects."

12. Do you enjoy working in a team?

Support what you say with examples so that the interviewer is convinced. Have at least three examples of working in different sized teams. Remember the P.E.E. (point, evidence, explanation) structure from Chapter 2.

The challenges in working in a small team (four members) are different to that of a bigger team (20 members). Try and use two contrasting examples to give a varied answer.

"I enjoy working in a team, and have worked in many different teams such as sports teams, the charity committee at school; where we raised money throughout the year for a charity of our choice; and through my work as a House Captain, which

included putting on our own production. What I enjoy most is seeing the end result of working together, as that sense of achievement shared within the group has always been second to none for me personally. "

13. Have you ever experienced death?

In answering a question like this the interview panel want to see your human side, and the thoughts you have surrounding death. Even though in medicine and dentistry, we are required to separate our emotions from our job, that's not to say we should not experience emotion at all. However, this is a very personal question and if you are uncomfortable sharing any personal experiences, you can simply let them know.

"I have experienced death in different ways. Firstly when I was 14, my cousin died following being found to have a brain tumour. As she had been an inpatient in hospital for a number of weeks, her death almost provided relief as we knew that she wasn't suffering anymore. Secondly, on my first day shadowing at a doctor at a hospital, a patient went into cardiac arrest and died in front of me, which was a traumatic experience to say the least. This was an interesting way to see death as it was at such close proximity, although I had neither seen nor interacted

with the patient, I was still quite taken aback by what had happened. And thirdly my grandfather a few months ago, which of the deaths I've experienced was the most difficult to cope with.

All three experiences were very different, but all of them they have made me appreciate life in a new way."

14. How do you deal with stress, as dentistry is a very long and stressful subject to study?

Keep this answer personal to you and demonstrate a well rounded appreciation of the demands of dentistry.

"I have a very strong support network of both friends and family who help me in times of stress by enabling me to talk about any problems I may be having. I have also found that exercise, and going for walks help me deal with stress."

15. Tell me about any of the situations where you have shown leadership skills.

Once again, refer back to the P.E.E. (point, evidence, explanation)structure to give a well rounded, yet unique answer.

"I used teamwork as well as leadership skills in my role as a House Captain, where I was responsible for producing and directing a theatre production. I had to audition people for roles, and allocate other people backstage roles. I would then oversee rehearsals, and liaise with the people responsible for costumes, music and stage props. As I was dealing with 15 girls between the ages of 11 and 17 I had to assert my authority at times. Thankfully the production was a success!

I look forward to building upon these skills at university in through new challenges. "

16. In ten years time after you have become a dentist and all your friends want to have a reunion but you are unable to attend, how would you want them to remember you?

"I would want them to remember me as a girl who got involved in all aspects of university life, who worked hard and played hard at appropriate times, and who made a significant contribution to some aspect of university life."

17. How can you relate being a dentist to playing competitive sport?

You can answer this using both positive and negative aspects of having competition in a workplace.

"I think every professional wants to be the top of their field, however, as in competitive sport this cannot be achieved alone. You need to be able to work with other members of your team, in this case other healthcare professionals to become the best you can be.

If you didn't do this in sport, you run the risk of losing the game; the equivalent of this in dentistry would be causing a problem, even death in a patient."

18. Have you ever considered taking a gap year?

"I considered it very briefly, but as I was keen to start university I decided I would rather travel after completing my education."

However, if you have taken a gap year that can be advantageous especially if you participated in some form of health care or volunteering, if so highlight in detail the nature of the work you did and how you feel it has made you a better medical candidate this time round.

19. What did you do for Duke of Edinburgh?

Try to highlight the points that display qualities that would be advantageous in dentistry, such as resilience, and ability to work in a team.

"For my Duke of Edinburgh, I travelled to Ecuador with a group of other students. While we were there we helped build a school, as well as 'buddying' up with an Ecuadorian person around the same age as ourselves, to help them improve their English. As the building project was led by us we had to work together to build it successfully.

Furthermore, we trekked through the Amazon, where teamwork was essential for us to avoid injury. This trek included scaling mountains, a difficult task for most but nearly impossible if one is afraid of height like me. However, due to resilience (and a lot of encouragement from my peers) I was able to reach the summit."

20. Have you ever had to make an unpopular decision as a leader?

Firstly explain your leadership role, and then detail the unpopular decision you made. If possible think of an unpopular decision that had gained you the respect of your peers and also turned out to be the correct decision for the situation.

"In my role as Deputy House Captain, we would hold events such as inter-house music competitions. Usually the final piece would be performed by one of the most talented musicians in the school, however I decided to break with tradition and perform a group number.

This was unpopular with not only other pupils performing in the show, but also the House Captain. This lead to a tense atmosphere in the lead up to the competition, but my decisions was proved correct when we won the competition and received a special commendation for our group performance."

21. Do you believe your communication and organisational skills are adequate to become a great dentist?

Never say yes, as these can always be improved upon...showing that you understand the need for continuous personal development.

"Although I feel I have very good communication and organisational skills, shown by previous roles I have held successfully such as House Captain while in Year 13, as well as participating heavily in church activities all the while without letting my academic standards slip; I feel that there is always more I can learn, and I hope that through experiences I hope to gain at dental school, my communication and organisation skills will develop further, therefore enabling me to eventually become a great dentist."

22. What would you describe as your worst qualities?

I would advise against putting anything down which would cause interview panels to look at you less favorably, such as being a pathological liar. With whatever bad quality you name try and show how it could be an advantage within dentistry, but what you could do to try and master it.

Examples:

Too nice: allow people to take me for granted

"One of my worst qualities is being too nice to everyone, as this allows people to take me for granted. However, I think that being too nice can certainly help you on the win over some of the more challenging patients. However, to improve this quality, I have tried to become more assertive, more vocal and less flexible when deemed necessary."

A perfectionist: always paying meticulous attention to detail

"I have often been told that I can spend far too long on even the simplest parts of a project as I am very keen to get it all perfectly as it should be. I am learning however that some tasks/projects require more time and attention and that I won't always be able to complete my assignments on time if I don't manage this better. I have started making lists in my diary and have allocated more time for projects that have a higher mark weighting. Hopefully, this method will also help me to be better organised while at university. "

23. How would your closest friends describe you?

In this answer, try to give a range of positives which would give the questioner a wider insight into your personality that you may not have showed already. Sound genuine and use specific, descriptive words with examples of why your friends would describe you in that way

"My closest friends would describe me as generous, as I am always willing to share what I have with them, loyal -as I will always be willing to stand by them in whatever they need help in doing and finally, organised, as I seem to be the one who always has to organize our social calender!"

24. How do you handle criticism?

No one likes criticism but it is a necessary part of life in order to improve and grow as a person. It would be easy to say "I love criticism! ... Give it to me all the time". However, honesty in these situations shows that you can truly reflect on your own character flaws (if you do have them). Think about why you dislike criticism (if you actually do like it – please ignore) and use it to construct your answer.

"As a proud person, I am sensitive to the criticism that I receive. However, I believe that feedback, positive or negative, is an integral part of improving myself when I received criticism I do attempt to understand why it is being said and further more question the source about ways I can improve that aspect of myself."

As this point it would also be appropriate to insert a real life experience, giving an example of when you have had to deal with critique.

25. Give me an example when you have had your opinions overridden, what did you do?

In scenario questions, there will always be situations that you may or may not have encountered. The most important thing is you think about the outcomes which would best reflect your character. If you are a strong willed person answer honestly however there is a fine line between trying to make your point heard and being argumentative. Come up with the most logical response so that it seems you are at least diplomatic in your thinking. However don't compromise your personality completely by being a 'push-over'.

"While in a committee meeting .... my point about changing X.... was disregarded by members of the committee, particularly the chair person, and although I tried to clarify my point, I believe that particularly when opposition for your idea comes from multiple sources it is important to re-evaluate whether your opinion is as valid as you think it was. Hence I took away the reasoning for the disagreement and came back in the next meeting with evidence for why I suggested such an action."

26. What person(s) has had the biggest positive impact on you?

This can be a personal question, however is a good opportunity to appreciate someone who has either inspired you through their words or actions as a role model, or someone who has directly contributed to your schooling or extra-curricular activities. Highlight the things you have learnt from them or how they have greatly affected your life. Finally talk about how you have taken it on board or how this impact will develop you as a person.

"My coach at my football club, Ridgeway Rovers FC

has been one of the most influential people in my life so far, over the last 2 years playing under his guidance, he has not only help me improved me as a footballer, but also instilled in me some of what he describes as the key values to succeeding in life. This includes hard work and dedication to your craft, making sure you are early to the things you need to be on time to, and finally having the confidence in yourself succeed in the task ahead of you.

These are some of the things which I have tried to apply not only to my sporting life, but more importantly to my personal and academic life and have helped me through much of my A levels so far."

27. How have you developed your communication skills?

The only way to develop your communication skills is to use your communication skills. Hence, before you can answer a question like this, you should have already been taking part in activities which will actually develop the skill of talking and listening effectively to people.

Activities such as taking part in debates, presentations, talks and public speaking help in showing that you have been able to display your communication skills. Meanwhile actively taking part in workshops, teaching sessions, and activity groups which focus on improving communications show that you have a keenness to improve.

Remember that almost every aspect of human life today requires good communication to be successful, so highlighting activities which shows your personal progression or improvement in your communication skills could be a more tactful way to answer a question like this.

The interviewers will immediately know from the first time you answer a question whether you have good communication skills, and so this is much more than a tick box exercise.

"Dentistry is about communication and so I strongly feel that one should think about developing one's communication skills constantly. I believe that these skills are the tools we are given to help carve out our future. Therefore, like any useful tool it needs to sharpened and kept ready to be used as any moment..."

28.Give examples of you showing that you have good dexterity?

Examples can range from art, instruments, designing models, woodwork to cake decorating or doing henna designs. Just anything that shows you working well with your hands, paying attention to detail within a confined space is adequate. Have at least 3 examples that you can talk about, if asked.

Chapter 7

WORK EXPERIENCE AND EDUCATION BASED QUESTIONS

1. How are your A-levels going?

2. How would any non-science subject at GCSE/A-level help as a dentist?

3. Which non-science subject that you have studied do you think will be useful in career in medicine and why?

4. Out of the work experience you have done what did you enjoy the most?

5. Tell us about your work experience?

6. What did you see in your work experience?

7. What did you dislike about your dentistry work experience?

8. What do you think are the main characteristics of a good dentist that you saw in practice?

9. In your work experience what is a problem a dentist found?

10. How would you handle a situation, where one of your patients has AIDS?

11. Is amalgam safe to use?

1. How are your A-levels going?

Not great? Is it a case of how would you LIKE your A-levels to be going? If they are going as well as you have hoped so far, say so and give the reasons why. However if they haven't been as straightforward as they could have been, make sure you sound positive or at the very least optimistic!! Again like with any question, giving examples is imperative.

"This year doing my A-levels has been the most challenging of my school life to date, with more independence over my learning while taking in new ideas and ways of thinking through the questions put to us, particularly in my science subjects. However it has also been enjoyable as I have been able to see myself grow as a person and become more responsible for my own learning and understanding. It has driven me to continue to work hard at the topics which I am weakest at!"

2. How would any non-science subject at GCSE/A-level help as a dentist?

Being a good dentist requires more than just scientific knowledge. As a dentist, you will play many roles; the communicator, the mediator, the presenter, the investigator. Therefore it is essential for any dentist to be versatile both in their skills and way of thinking.

That is why doing non-science subject at GSCE and A levels can be a great benefit in developing more than just your scientific skills. Subjects like History, Law and Criminology help to critically analyse sources, while Psychology and Sociology help us understand human behaviours.

They can all play a part in shaping you as a doctor so don't be afraid to admit your interest in the different subjects that you have taken as long as you can justify how it can help mould you into the best possible dentist you can be...

"As a dentist, I believe you need to be a well-rounded and conscientious individual in order to have perspective on some of the major clinical decisions which you will be taking, which can have huge implications on the lives of the patients who you treat. Hence I believe that having knowledge and experience of alternative subjects which broaden the way that you interpret and understand the world

beneficial.

Having studied Psychology at A level myself, I have found myself being able to look at the effect of the brain on our relationships and our illnesses. It has made me appreciate how Biology and Chemistry doesn't always explain the things that we do as concisely as we're taught to believe!"

Once again give examples of how you have personally tried to achieve what you are describing

3. Which non-science subject that you have studied do you think will be useful in career in medicine and why?

This is your opportunity to explore abstract ideas about how your favorite subjects could potentially help you to become the best dentist you could be!

However keep the weird and wonderful connections to within reason and build a solid case for the subject with 3 key points to justify why you think that subject will be useful in a dental career.

"Having studied Electronics at GSCE, I believe that it will benefit me in a future surgical career within dentistry. Firstly, while learning the basic principles of building electrical circuits, the most important skill I learnt was comprehensive planning and improving my manual skills.

In order to build a working circuit, all the possibilities must be thought of in advance with calculations of what capacitors; resistors and etc. are needed before a wire is laid out.

This is similar to any good surgeon's routine whereby the right equipment and method must be thought out well in advance. Secondly, in order to have a complete working circuit, vigorous testing and review of your work in progress is needed, something which every surgeon should be considering as he is carrying out any procedure.

Finally, in Electronics class we were taught that although circuitry is important, presentation is equally as important in ensuring user friendliness. Similarly surgeons are always required to think about aesthetics of their finished procedure in order to satisfy patients."

4. Out of the work experience you have done what did you enjoy the most?

Work experience is one of the most important components of the dental student application and although is mandatory should still be relatively enjoyable! Even if it was the most boring thing you've ever done, try to take any positives that you can from your work experience to be able to sell yourself, but most importantly sell the experience to the interviewers as one that has made you a better candidate to get into dental school.

If you truly have had an awesome experience in your work experience, really sell it and show your enthusiasm, and as with any question, bring the example you give to life!

Talk about the state of the art equipment you saw, the way in which the dentist interacted with his team and the patient and dealt with anxiety.

"I thoroughly enjoyed my placement at Plaistow Dental surgery. It was interesting to see how the dentist dealt with anxiety at different levels in different patients. It became evident to me that this was a barrier to providing efficient dental care and

109

dentists all over have different ways to approach the situation. In addition, I deeply admired the craftsmanship and agility required to perform some of the procedures and the way in which the procedures were explained to the patient, in simple and generic terms.

The dentist explained some of the techniques of local anaesthesia which encompassed different nerve root blocks and what can happen if this went wrong. I found this entire experience both mentally stimulating and physically challenging."

5. Tell us about your work experience?

This should be straight forward as you would have done loads and loads of different and varied work experience placements to broaden your horizons and learn a bit more about the field of medicine... Although this would be the ideal situation, work experience in a healthcare environment has become an even more difficult goal to achieve due to increases in health and safety regulations and increased scrutiny in healthcare environments. However it is important that whatever work experience placement you have a clear structure for answering the question:

Where it was: in a hospital/clinic/surgery environment, although if this is not possible, just justify any location by what you gained from the experience as explained below...

How you obtained it: Self organised placements with a good back story always show your perseverance

What did you do?: Assisting in surgery or looking after patients can look glamorous but is difficult to get to do, so working in a more administrative role may not be as fun, but can be reflected on.

Who did you encounter? : Dentists (who can give you advice), Patients (who you enjoy spending time with and learning from) and other professionals (which helps you understand roles with the healthcare team)

What did you learn?: This is by far the most important part of the answer, as it will show the interviewers how reflective you are as an individual and whether you have the right attitude and aptitude to be a dental student.

6. What did you see in your work experience?

This is a chance to really express your interest in what you saw and what further cemented your passion to do dentistry. Take the time to talk about where you went and why, how long for, what you saw, how it was done, how long it took, what instruments were used, what discussions were had with the patient. Know some of the procedures you saw in detail and be ready to explain what happened step by step for these procedures; (e.g. informed patient of treatment they needed and patient consented-used local anaesthetic-checked the patient was numb with a sharp probe-placed rubber dam with a clamp etc) It's also helps to know why each part was done.

"I did my work experience in at Hospital in London and at one of the practices I applied to nearer to my home, for a total of 6 weeks to gain further understanding of dentistry in general practice and in a hospital environment. This was a truly invaluable experience. I saw a range of treatments in the hospital particularly emergency extractions which were very exciting, what I liked the most about this environment was how some patients would arrive in severe pain affecting their sleep and leave in a much better state than when they arrived. In general practice I really enjoyed the relationship the dentist had with their patient. The dentist was very hard

working and carried out a broad range of treatments from fillings to taking impressions for dentures or crowns. They worked very well with their team of fellow dentists, nurses and receptionists, I really admired this."

7. What did you dislike about your dentistry work experience?

It's okay to dislike some things but they do have to be rational. Avoid disliking anything directly about dentistry as it doesn't look very good to already be disliking things about dentistry before properly learning about it. As well as that if there is something you did dislike, try to talk about how you are working around this dislike or how you've come to understand more about it or no longer dislike it.

"I initially disliked getting up so early every morning to travel so far for work experience. I managed to acclimatise to this but the first couple of days were challenging. With regards to the dentist it was an eye opener to see that sometimes they would work right through lunch and only have a few minutes to have some food. When things are busy, or overrun, or time is tight this is something that may have to happen and this is true of most jobs so it's just something to also be prepared for."

8. What do you think are the main characteristics of a good dentist that you saw in practice?

Not only do they want to see that you know some of the characteristics that make a good dentist, they want to know that you were actively observing these qualities and seeing WHY they are good characteristics in practice and how it helped the patient or the dentist or the practice as a whole.

"The dentist I worked with had great interpersonal skills, they communicated effectively with their patients so they understood and were comfortable with treatment they were having, they also listened very well to gain better understanding of patients symptoms and expectations of treatment. They worked well with their nurse, as well as their receptionist and fellow dentists. It's important to have these skills because they are pivotal to having a friendly and comfortable environment for patients and staff. The dentist was a very good leader and it appeared that the practice was run very well because each member was aware of their roles and the tasks they had to do on a day to day basis. The dentist thought well on his, because they would tell me after certain procedures that had not gone to plan, what they did to amend the unexpected changed e.g. losing more than expected of the tooth when doing a filling."

9. In your work experience what is a problem a dentist found?

This is a simple question to talk further about what you observed on work experience. Once the problem has been talked about, thinks about how the dentist got around or fixed this problem. Try to think of how the problem may have been avoided in the first place or better managed to show you are thinking beyond the scope of the question.

"In my work experience in general practice the dentist I observed had problems with a crown that came back from the lab. It did not fit properly and they were not happy to cement that crown down there and then. After the appointment over lunch they phoned the lab to speak to the technician who made the crown and told them the problems with the crown. They agreed on a way to make it fit better and the crown was sent back and fixed to be fitted at a later date. Unfortunately I was unable to see the second fitting but they told me it was fine. I think a way to have avoided this would be clear instruction to the lab if the crown is going to be a tricky one, or maybe phone the lab before the crown is made to explain any fine details to do with the crown."

10.How would you handle a situation, where one of your patients has AIDS?

The infection control policies used in dentistry are designed to minimise the transfer of infection from patient to dentist and vice versa. The phrase 'Treat everybody as they might have a transmittable infection, because they may not know themselves' leaves the dentist and patient safe in almost any scenario. The dentist must wear gloves, apron, mask and goggles to protect them, while the patient wears glasses and an apron also.

"I think hospitals have infection control procedures that cover patients with any transmittable infections. As long as there are reasonable precautions in place there is no reason why a patient with AIDS should not be treated. On my work experience the dentist treated a HIV positive patient just like any other because he had protective clothing on."

11.Is amalgam safe to use?

Amalgam (while it's use is reducing) is safe to use on patients which is why the UK government has not yet removed it from NHS practice. The mercury u amalgam is in minute doses when being placed in the mouth and then is inert once the amalgam is set. When being removed there is a risk of a very small dose of mercury being absorbed by the patient and the dentist but with adequate suction and safety this can be avoided. It is likely to be removed in future do to environmental problems with its disposal. (It needs to be stored in cold water and disposed of by relevant companies safely as opposed to just being thrown away). A large amount of mercury inappropriately disposed of in the environment is obviously not ideal.

NOTES

Chapter 8

DENTAL & INDUSTRY BASED QUESTIONS

1. Do you think pharmacists are sometimes tempted to tell a customer to buy an expensive product even if there is a cheaper one available?

2. Dentists use a lot of materials in their daily practice for several procedures. Do you know of any materials? What properties do you think they require?

3. What is gum disease? What are the consequences if left untreated?

4. Who gets Gum disease?

5. What is plaque?

6.Why do you think women with periodontal disease have an increased risk of having premature babies? *Note this is an unlikely question, but is here to remind you to think scientifically*

7.Early Childhood carries (ECC) is a damaging form of dental decay, which affects the teeth of pre-schoolers. What preventative measures do you think could help avoid this.

8. Oral Hygiene is of utmost importance in the field of dentistry. What would you do to promote oral hygiene

for your patients?

9. What according to you is the best brushing technique?

10. Can you expand on oral hygiene aids?

11. What do you know about the effects of smoking on dental health?

12. What are dental caries and what foods make it worse?

13. What do you think are the five most common dental complaints?

14. What is oral cancer?

15. How Is Oral Cancer Diagnosed?

16. How do you go about keeping up to date with current dental issues?

17. How do you think dentists are viewed in the current media?

18. How does a dentist promote good health?

1. Do you think pharmacists are sometimes tempted to tell a customer to buy an expensive product even if there is a cheaper one available?

This is a circumstantial question so you have to weight up both arguments for and against even if you believe, and perhaps know what the answer is, as you cannot afford to generalise. Be honest with yourself and the interviewer if you don't have as much of a perspective on a circumstance as this shows your honesty and if possible, offer to try and improve yourself by wanting to find out. Also feel free to provide your own personal commentary as long as you distinguish it as your own opinion.

"I think that there may be some pharmacists, who may be tempted to sell more expensive polyproducts that may also be of better or more proven quality and so the sale of it is still justified. I think that a problem with commercialising healthcare will always causes dilemmas such as this, as when should the healthcare provider stop being a seller and vice versa. I don't know if pharmacists have the same duty to their patients as doctors and dentists do, however, it would be nice to know that pharmacists care about the wellbeing of their customers and would not just sell products to make money, but also to ensure that they are doing the best for their health."

2. Dentists use a lot of materials in their daily practice for several procedures. Do you know of any materials? What properties do you think they require?

The properties of dental materials can be classified as being mechanical (strength), physical (thermal expansion), chemical (corrosion) and biocompatibility (toxicity). Furthermore, they can also be defined by their molecular form; metals, polymers, ceramics and composites. Dental amalgam is an alloy of silver and tin and resin composites are another example of a commonly used material.

Some of the mechanical properties that the material should possess or be considered include that of stress, strain, elastic deformation, plastic deformation, brittleness, ductility, hardness ,strength etc.

Some of the physical properties to consider include electrical conductivity, thermal conductivity, thermal expansion, radio- opacity and optical properties.

In addition, chemical properties include corrosion, solubility and formation of an oxide layer. (Note all metals – except noble ,metals like gold , form an oxide layer on the metal surface; this can either be uneven and porous or uniform, tightly bound and non-porous.)

Basic theory is that dental materials should not be carcinogenic (the ability of a substance to induce uncontrolled division of other cells –cancer), not readily induce hypersensitivity reactions and not produce systemic toxic effects. This is because the materials will be in contact with the patient for a prolonged period of time and any material that causes harm is

3. What is gum disease? What are the consequences if left untreated?

Gum disease (periodontal disease) is a chronic infection (occurring over a long period of time unlike an acute infection – which has a sudden onset) most commonly resulting from a buildup of dental plaque. Research has linked gum disease to an array of other medical conditions such as pneumonia and chronic respiratory disease, heart disease etc. However, gum disease only shows signs and symptoms once it's in its advanced stages.

Gingivitis is a mild form of gum disease that can usually be reversed with daily brushing and flossing, and regular cleaning by a dentist or dental hygienist.

This differs from more severe forms of gum disease where one could lose bone and connective tissue which hold teeth in place. Instead, it is characterized by gums that are red, swollen and prone to bleed easily. However, when gingivitisis is left untreated, it can progress to periodontitis (inflammation around the tooth).

In periodontitis, gums have the tendency to haul away from the teeth and form spaces (called "pockets") that then go on to become infected. The body's immune system targets these bacteria as the plaque spreads and grows below the gum line. The body's immune system acts to break down the bone and connective tissue that hold teeth in place. If then left untreated the bones, gums, and connective tissue are completely destroyed. This eventually results is loose teeth which then have to be extracted.

4. Who gets Gum disease?

Gum disease is resultant of plaque buildup underneath the gum line. This buildup is gradual and therefore the signs of it are seen later, usually when people are in their 30s or 40s. Overall, it is thought that men are more likely to have gum disease than women.

Teenagers on the other hand, rarely develop periodontitis, they can however develop gingivitis, the milder form of gum disease. An early sign of this is bleeding gums whilst brushing.

Anyone with less than average standards of dental hygiene can get gum disease but there are certain risk factors that increase your chances of contracting the disease. These include the following:

Smoking- Smoking is one of the most significant risk factors associated with the development of gum disease. Furthermore, smoking can lower the chances for successful treatment.

Hormonal imbalances in girls/women- These changes can make gums more sensitive and make it easier for gingivitis to develop.

Diabetes- Patients with diabetes are at higher risk for developing infections, including gum disease.

Other illnesses- Diseases like cancer or AIDS, which attacks the body's immune defenses and their treatments (e.g. chemotherapy) again which can kill healthy cells can also negatively affect the health of gums.

Medications- There are hundreds of prescription and over the counter medications that can reduce the flow of saliva, which has a protective effect on the mouth. The lack of saliva makes the mouth vulnerable to infections such as gum disease. Meanwhile, some medicines can accelerate abnormal growth of the gum tissue; making it that much more difficult to maintain clean teeth and gums (always read side effects of prescriptions)

Genetic susceptibility- Some people are more prone to severe gum disease than others, as a result of inherited traits.

5. What is plaque?

Dental plaque consists of a colourless film of bacteria. This plaque coats one's teeth and easily gets between the tooth surface and the actual gum tissue. Over time , the plaque hardens into tarter (also known as calculus) and causes the gums to become inflamed. If left untreated, the inflammation can develop into a serious infection, attacking the bone that supports the teeth and causing the gum to shrink.

6. Why do you think women with periodontal disease have an increased risk of having premature babies? *Note this is an unlikely question, but is here to remind you to think scientifically*

There are two possibilities. Firstly, the toxins that enter the bloodstream through the inflamed gums separating from the bone may create stress for the foetus, which in turn may lead to a premature birth. Secondly, the bacteria associated with gum disease may work to boost the hormone, prostaglandin- which stimulates labour.

7. Early Childhood carries (ECC) is a damaging form of dental decay, which affects the teeth of pre-schoolers. What preventative measures do you think could help avoid this.

Early childhood carries could lead to further dental decay and this could have a detrimental impact on young children as it would cause them pain, loss of appetite and lack of sleep. Therefore, if measures could be taken to reduce this, it would prove beneficial to both parents and the children. Good dental habits are key even as a toddler, possibly preventing the baby from falling asleep with a bottle of juice or milk in his/her mouth, cleaning the mouth with a damp cloth after feeding etc are measures that can be taken to reduce the likelihood of ECC.

8. Oral Hygiene is of utmost importance in the field of dentistry. What would you do to promote oral hygiene for your patients?

Think of innovative ways to highlight the importance of oral hygiene to the patient. Simply telling them to brush their teeth might not be enough in this instance.

" If I was a dentist and I had to promote oral hygiene within my practice, I would firstly have animated videos with the importance of oral hygiene playing on the screens in the waiting rooms, so patients of all ages can view them and adhere to tips easily. I'd also hand out leaflets to patients reminding them of the most effective brushing technique with vivid images and little text, so that it appeals to them. Finally, if patients still are reluctant to comply, I could help them visualize the plaque by enhancing it using disclosing agents and then showing them using a hand held mirror"

9. What according to you is the best brushing technique?

There are numerous techniques for you to find. But of these the modified Bass Technique is the simplest and most effective. Here the head of the toothbrush should be angled so that the filaments are at 45° to the long axis of the tooth and should be placed at the gum margin so that the filaments can enter the gingival crevice. Then a back and forth movement should be used to facilitate plaque removal. But another technique called the Charter's Technique is used in patients with braces. Here you almost clean sections around each bracket at a time, aiming to remove as much debris and associated bacteria with it.

10. Can you expand on oral hygiene aids?

Successful prevention and treatment of periodontal disease is heavily dependent on the ability of a patient to maintain an adequate standard of plaque control.

Oral hygiene aids are vital to ensure good dental hygiene and as dentists, the earlier you instil them in your patients, the better their teeth life will be. Examples are toothbrushes, manual and electric for those with reduced manual dexterity, floss – either waxed or unwaxed, tape- broader than floss, superfloss – used for cleaning under bridge pontics and wooden sticks.

11. What do you know about the effects of smoking on dental health?

Cigarette smoking is a significant risk factor for two main dental conditions, namely, periodontitis and ANUG (acute necrotizing ulcerative gingivitis). Several mechanisms have been suggested as to how smoking predisposes to periodontal disease. The vasoconstrictive effect of nicotine may interfere with the host response mechanisms. Smoking may also influence the microbial composition of dental plaque. Patients who smoke are 4 times more likely to develop periodontitis. Therefore, it must be remembered that as a dental student and future dentist, you must always encourage patients to quit smoking. Stopping smoking benefits periodontal health and improves the outcome of treatment.

The four A's Smoking cessation routine, originally devised in the US is a useful aid.

ASK- all patients about smoking

ADVICE- all smokers about the benefits of quitting

ASSIST- those patients who express an interest in stopping, either formally or by referring them to a smoking cessation

ARRANGE- follow- up visits

12. What are dental caries and what foods make it worse?

Dental caries, otherwise also known as tooth decay is a bacterial infection which results in demineralisation and eventual destruction of the hard surfaces such as dentin (on teeth). This occurs as a result of bacterial fermentation of the food debris that accumulates on the teeth.

It has been shown that caries does not develop in germ-free animals, even when fed a carcinogenic diet. Therefore, caries results not from a single bacterial species but by the acid production of a range of organisms. Some examples of organisms causing dental caries include Mutans streptococci and lactobacillus species.

Carbohydrates that can be easily metabolized by oral bacteria are an essential necessity for caries development. These include sugars from whole fruits and vegetables ; mainly fructose, glucose and sucrose and sugars from milk and milk containing products; lactose etc. There is extensive evidence of the correlation between the frequency and amount of sugar consumption and the prevalence and severity of dental caries.

13. What do you think are the five most common dental complaints?

Bad Breath (or halitosis) is one of the most common dental health issues. Brushing and flossing regularly can help avoid this problem but most of the time if it persists there may be a suggestive underlying dental cause.

Cavities or dental caries are another most commonly viewed problem in the UK. This is a result of a combination of acidic environment (plaque combined with food) and sugars on the dentin and enamel of teeth. Avoiding or reducing one's sugar intake and sticking with healthy foods can minimize the risk of tooth decay.

Gum disease is an infection in the periodontal (gum) tissue surrounding your teeth, and is the leading cause of tooth loss in adults. The early stages of gum disease, known as gingivitis, can usually be treated easily. Advanced stages of gum disease, or periodontitis, may require surgery to correct. If you have bright or inflamed gums, contact your dentist, as gum disease has been clinically linked to heart attacks and stroke.

cold sores, ulcers, fever blisters, and thrush are not bothersome and uncomfortable, they can be signs of a more serious problem. Mouth sores that remain for over two weeks can be indicative of a more serious dental problem.

Oral cancer is a serious dental disease which affects millions of people world-wide and hundreds of thousands of new cases are diagnosed every year. Most oral cancers can quickly spread through your mouth. Most cases of oral cancer are related to the use of smoking, tobacco, and alcohol. Human papillomavirus infection (HPV), irritation of your gum tissue (such as that cause by dentures or a filling), and poor dental hygiene have also been linked to the onset of oral cancer. Studies show that men are twice as likely as women to get oral cancer. This very serious dental disease can affect the mouth, lips, and/or throat, but thanks to early diagnosis and treatment by your dentist it is highly curable with very positive recovery chances.

" I think the most common reasons for patients' visits to dentists are tooth pain as a result of numerous dental caries, bleeding gums as a result of gum disease; either gingivitis in a young person or

periodontitis in an older person, cold sores or swellings in the mouth. Other common complaints could include bad breath (Halitosis) that hasn't gone away even after trying measures of chewing gum and mouthwash etc. I am basing these cases on the most frequent visit to dentists I had myself and on accounts of what I witnessed during my work experience"

14. What is oral cancer?

Cancer itself is defined as the uncontrollable growth of cells that invade and cause damage to surrounding tissue. Oral cancer or mouth cancer appears as a growth or sore in the mouth that persists despite remedies. It can affect the tongue and lips more commonly that other parts. However, it can also affect the cheeks (buccal lining), floor of the mouth (lingual surface) , hard and soft palate, sinuses, and throat (pharynx) .Like most cancers, oral cancer can be life threatening if not diagnosed and treated early.

According to the American Cancer Society, men face twice the risk of developing oral cancer as women, and men who are over age 50 face the greatest risk. It's estimated that over 35,000 people in the U.S. received a diagnosis of oral cancer in 2008.

Risk factors for the development of oral cancer include:

Smoking - Cigarette, cigar, or pipe smokers are six times more likely than non smokers to develop oral cancers.

Smokeless tobacco users- Users of dip, snuff, or chewing tobacco products are 50 times more likely to develop cancers of the cheek, gums, and lining of the lips.

Excessive consumption of alcohol- Oral cancers are about six times more common in drinkers than in non drinkers.

Family history of cancer.

Excessive sun exposure- especially at a young age.

It is important to note that over 25% of all oral cancers occur in people who do not smoke and who only drink alcohol occasionally.

15. How Is Oral Cancer Diagnosed?

As a dentist you will conduct routine oral cancer screening exams on patients that you see regularly. The main thing of interest is to feel for any lumps or irregular tissue changes in the patient's neck, head, face, and oral cavity. Inside the mouth, as a dentist and therefore dental student, you should look for any sores or discoloured tissue as well as check for any signs and symptoms mentioned above.

If something does seem irregular, the dentist can perform a small procedure called a brush biopsy. This test is painless and involves taking a small sample of the tissue and analyzing it for abnormal cells. Alternatively, if the tissue looks more complex, your dentist may recommend a scalpel biopsy, a procedure usually carried out under requires local anaesthetic. These tests play a crucial role in helping to detect oral cancer early, before it has had a chance to progress and spread to other organs etc.

16. How do you go about keeping up to date with current dental issues?

This question is asking how do you show your interest in the field of dentistry through reading, and it is important to show that you do so via a variety of reliable methods. Always be prepared to talk about a current article you may have seen from the sources you mentioned.

Newspapers although good for reading, lack concrete scientific grounding, often paraphrasing from real science to fit their purpose.

Magazines such as New Scientist are well rounded scientific publications which help broaden your knowledge of science around the world.

The internet is the main source of information in the

world today, many websites have health sections such as the BBC, while you can search for numerous scientific journals and abstracts in the fields which you are interested in.

"I usually keep up to date with current dental issues via a number of ways. I try to keep up daily by visiting a website called dentistrytoday.com which collates sources from a variety of journals such as the BDJ as well as other news sources to deliver dental news, it is usually the first place I go to read about developments in, while I also use the BBC Health website to look at more British focused news articles. Furthermore I subscribe to the New Scientist magazine, which I find to be a really good read, updating me on current medical, dental and scientific news while having a range of interesting articles."

17. How do you think dentists are viewed in the current media?

Negative high profile stories about dentists are always going to be around as the media always focus on the negatives and less on the positives particularly in professions or fields where they feel people are highly paid compared to the general population. Use this question to demonstrate your knowledge of recent dental stories which involve dentists to impress the interviewers.

"I think that the current media viewpoint of dentists is not positive, especially as they often like to focus on the stories of individual dentists who may not be doing good things. I read a recent Telegraph article on the internet about a dentist who in the recent strike, cancelled his NHS clinic due to strike action, but however was not too far away doing paid work at a private hospital. Stories like that affect public confidence in dentists, and with high profile stories such as Harold Shipman and Andrew Wakefield, it seems that the media will take any opportunity to bring down the medical/ dental profession. Despite this, I think the one medium which is very sympathetic to doctors is television, with programmes like 24hours in A&E and Junior Doctors. But I think it's about time to make one for dentists too"

18. How does a dentist promote good health?

Here it is important to know how to promote good oral health beyond simply brushing twice a day. With dentistry now in a minimally invasive and preventative ethos (and the 2014 NHS contract that appears to have this as the focus as opposed to units of dental activity) it is vital that you are aware of ways of preventing oral disease and promoting good health.

Oral Hygiene- Brush x2/day (at night and one other time of the day for at least 2 minutes) with a fluoride toothpaste (1450ppm for adults 1000ppm for under 6's) medium-soft brush. All surfaces of the teeth should be brushed with a Modified Bass technique (or any technique that does not cause damage but removes plaque effectively. Effective plaque removal can help prevent tooth decay and gum disease. Flossing once a day or using interdental brushes is also vital for effective plaque removal.

Fluoride- this is an element that inhibits enzymes in the bacteria in plaque thus preventing them metabolising carbohydrates and producing acids that demineralise teeth and cause tooth decay. It also hardens the enamel and makes it more acid resistant by binding to it. Fluoride is available in a variety of ways (toothpaste, mouthrinses, tablets, varnishes, water supply)-KNOW AREAS IN THE UK THAT CURRENTLY HAVE FLUORIDATED WATER SUPPLY-NEWCASTLE, BIRMINGHAM AND AREAS THAT ARE NOT-LONDON, BATH AND AREAS UNDER DEBATE-SOUTHAMPTON

Toothpaste and mouthrinses are the most commonly used dentrifices for patients at home. A dentist may place fluoride varnish or prescribe tablets for higher risk patients or use the varnish to prevent any problems arising if potential for future high risk is likely.

Diet Advice- high sugar diets (carbonated drinks, sweets, crisps etc) help plaque bacteria flourish and produce more acid to cause tooth decay. Dentists should advise patients to lower the frequency of sugary foods and drinks they have so as to reduce the number of acid attacks on their teeth, if they are going to eat them to have them at meal times.

Scale and Polish- This treatment can be provided by a dentist using ultrasonic and hand scalers to remove calculus (mineralised hardened plaque that is very difficult for the patient to otherwise remove). This s helpful as plaque sticks to calculus and can cause further problems (particularly gum disease) for the patient.

Provide smoking cessation advice-smoking is strongly linked to gum disease with 40-50% of smokers having some form of gum disease. It is important to warn patients that smoking will not only increase their chance of having gum disease but will also reduce their chance of responding well to treatment for gum disease.

Regular reviews of the advice given-patients should attend the dentist every 6 months to ensure they have taken all the health promotion advice on board and have not developed tooth decay or gum disease-if they have developed them regular visits allows them to be spotted early and treated effectively.

"A dentist can and should promote oral health to all of their patients, especially to the patients that are high risk (high number of cavities or fillings/crowns). A patient should be warned of the consequences of bad oral hygiene (gun disease and tooth decay .

This involves advice on oral hygiene and how to clean their teeth with the right kind of brush and fluoride toothpaste and flossing also, they should advice the patient on the use of fluoride and its benefits. Diet advice may be necessary if patients are higher risk so they are aware of foods that are good and bad for their teeth. If the patient has hardened calculus that is difficult to remove present in their mouth a scale and polish is a good way to give the patient cleansable teeth again to help them avoid gum disease. If the patient smokes smoking cessation advice should be given because of the high correlation in smoking and gum disease. This advice should be regularly reviewed with the patient via repeated check-ups every 6 months to ensure it has been taken on board and any disease that develops is spotted and treated early and effectively"

Chapter 9

DENTISTRY IN THE NHS

We will keep this chapter short and concise. When you sit your dental school interviews it is unlikely you will be asked complex or detailed questions about the National Health Service (NHS). This is a knowledge you will develop over your undergraduate training and once you are out within practice in your foundation training year. Our advice is not to try and learn everything possible about NHS Dentistry; there is a lot and it can get confusing. Focus on understanding the main principles, mechanisms and payment options in order to be able to answer the standard of question that will be asked.

Some of this has been covered in other chapters but to recap let us start with the background of the NHS.

The NHS was founded on July 5th 1948 by Aneurin Bevan, the Health Secretary at the time. His plan was to for the first time, bring hospitals, doctors, nurses, pharmacists, opticians and dentists together under one umbrella organization to provide services that are free for all at the point of delivery.

Aneurin believed good healthcare should be available to all, regardless of wealth, a core principle which is upheld to this day. Healthcare is financed entirely from taxation, which means people pay according to what is feasible for them.

However there are three services that are not free at the point of delivery. They are:

Prescriptions

Optical services

Dental Services

So whilst the NHS is a publically funded health service, your role as a dentist will not be directly comparable to that of your medical colleagues.

There is a yearly NHS budget which is allocated at different percentages to all the different fields under the umbrella. For 2012 to 2013 this budget was set by Parliament at £108.9 billion. You can look online for percentage breakdowns if this is something you are interested in, but you will unlikely be asked on it.

A useful website for you to use at this stage is the NHS Choices website which outlines the NHS, its set up, principles and treatment available for the general public. It concisely and explains everything and may help answer any questions you have.

Example Questions

Can you summarise your understanding of Dentistry within the NHS?

"The NHS is one the largest publically funded healthcare services. Set up in 1948 by Aneurin Bevan, its core principle was and still is to provide quality healthcare to all, regardless of their wealth, with payment through taxation.

For medical services it allows treatment and care to be provided without payment at the point of delivery. However dental care is an exception to this and patients are charged at the time of their appointments."

Can patients receive any treatment they want under the NHS?

The NHS states that:

'All the treatment that your dentist believes is necessary to achieve and maintain good oral health is available on the NHS. This means that the NHS provides any treatment you need to keep your mouth, teeth and gums healthy and free of pain.'

There can often be a dispute over cosmetic work being available under the NHS, for example white (composite) fillings. If a tooth needs a filling and the best option for the tooth is a white filling then this is deemed acceptable. This may be the case if the tooth is at the front of the mouth and having a silver (amalgam) filling could cause psychological or emotional stress for the patient as aesthetically the filling is visible at all times and not pleasing if in silver.

Another common misconception is that implants are not available under the NHS. Again if for example there is a medical condition, out of the patients control, which has caused loss of the teeth and there is NO other viable replacement option (dentures, bridges etc) then implants may be advocated.

The key to understanding what is available is the last sentence of the above quote: anything that is needed to keep the mouth 'healthy' and 'free of pain'; not necessarily what looks best.

146

An example answer could include:

"As I understand, the guidelines set out by the NHS stipulate that 'the treatment available to patients under the NHS is that which is required to keep their mouth, teeth and gums healthy and free of pain'. In some cases, the best solution to adhere to this is also an aesthetically pleasing one, in some cases it is not. It is down to the dentist's clinical judgment to decide what the best solution is from their training and other guidelines set out.

In an ideal world, we would want to be able to give the patients all treatment they desire but with a fixed NHS budget this is not possible and priority must go to treating that which is unhealthy as opposed to that which is healthy but could be improved."

Do you know anything about the current NHS contract?

"The current dental contract was introduced in 2006. It works through 'Units of Dental Activity' (UDAs). Each dentist/practice is allocated a number of UDAs which they must fulfil within the year. Each UDA has a financial value associated with it and when the units are achieved this value is received by the dentist/practice. If a dentist does not reach their

target they can be penalised financially. If they exceed their targets they do not earn extra."

How do the different treatment options available to the public relate to these Units of Dental Activity (UDAs)?

This is a breakdown of what number of UDAs each dentist/practice receives for certain treatments:

<u>One UDA</u> (also known as a Band 1 course of treatment)
This covers an examination, diagnosis (including X-rays), advice on how to prevent future problems, a scale and polish if needed, and application of fluoride varnish or fissure sealant.

<u>Three UDAs</u> (also known as a Band 2 course of treatment)
This covers everything listed in Band 1 above, plus any further treatment such as fillings, root canal work or removal of teeth.

<u>Twelve UDAs</u> (also known as a Band 3 course of treatment)
This covers everything listed in Bands 1 and 2 above, plus crowns, dentures and bridges.

Do patients pay for NHS dental treatment?

"Yes, they do pay for NHS dental treatment. The NHS is funded through taxation and for the large amount of services available; there is no payment at the point of delivery. However dental services, alongside optical services and prescriptions are an exception to this. There is a payment required at the time of the appointment.

Charges are related to the UDAs/Bands of treatment (see above).

For a Band 1 treatment the patient pays £18.00

For a Band 2 treatment the patient pays £49.00

For a Band 3 treatment the patient pays £214.00

An exception to this is if a patient attends without a pre-booked appointment/with an appointment booked on the day for emergency care whereby the patient will only pay a Band 1 charge of treatment (£18.00) regardless of what treatment is required."

Is any dental treatment free?

"Yes, you do not have to pay a dental charge:

to have your dentures repaired (sometimes it's not possible to repair dentures and a new denture may be required, which you would need to pay for as a Band 3 charge) , for having stitches out , if your dentist has to stop bleeding from your mouth , if your dentist only needs to write a prescription, although if you pay for prescriptions you will still need to pay the usual charge when you collect your medicine from your pharmacist"

If the NHS is funded by taxation and patients need to pay for dental treatment, what happens to those patients who are not currently being taxed?

"In these situations there are certain 'exemptions' or 'allowances' made for these patients. The following patients will not need to pay for treatment at the point of delivery:

Anyone aged under 18

Anyone under 19 and receiving full-time education

Anyone pregnant or has had a baby in the previous

12 months

Anyone staying in an NHS hospital and the treatment is carried out by the hospital dentist

An NHS hospital dental service outpatient (however, you may have to pay for your dentures or bridges).

Anyone on Income Support

Anyone on Income-related Employment and Support Allowance

Anyone on Income-based Jobseeker's Allowance

Anyone on Pension Credit guarantee credit

If you are named on a valid NHS tax credit exemption certificate or you are entitled to an NHS tax credit exemption certificate"

Are there any current changes happening in NHS Dentistry that you know about?

Since September 2011, there has been a new NHS contract being piloted by roughly 70 practices all over the UK with the aim to have it in place across all practices for April 2014. Previous to the pilot, the Department of Health looked at certain parameters such as access and quality of care for patients and overall improvements in the public's oral health and realised that with certain adjustments and a new

151

contract we could further improve these parameters.

The aims and objectives of the contract are to:

Promote prevention

Focus on improving the populations oral health – not just 'fix the problem when it happens'

To improve access, reduce inequalities and use the whole team to deliver care

The way it is put into place is detailed, with many clinical pathways. If asked a question of this nature in your interview use it to show you are keeping up to date on changes that will be in place by the time you qualify but you do not need to know details about how the pilot specifically runs so do not get bogged down with these. Just understand what it is trying to achieve – to improve the population's oral health through preventing the problem.

A model answer could include:

"Through the news and my own research I have been interested to see that there is a new dental contract pilot taking place over the UK. This contract which has been piloted so far by 70 UK practices started in September 2011 and is still ongoing. The aim is to improve the oral health of the population with emphasis on preventing disease rather than managing it once it has occurred. The Department of Health seem keen to have patients involved in the

care of their mouth as well as the dentists and have introduced incentives into the contract to get patients to do so. By using a 'RAG' scoring system:

RED – Stop, you need to take more care and have some treatment

AMBER – You could benefit from a little help from us

GREEN – You are doing well

they can show patients where their oral health stands and discuss what needs to be done to improve it through patient actions and dentists actions."

On your application I can see that you did some work experience in an NHS practice and a private practice. What differences did you observe and which did you prefer?

Try to give a balanced answer here. You can give an opinion at the end if you feel you preferred one over the other but remember to justify it.

For example:

"My work experience in the NHS showed me just how much we are able to offer patients under the public

health system. The days I spent there were fast-paced, and fully-booked with a turnover of around fifteen to twenty patients a day. I noticed that many of the patients attending for assessments were in pain or required a lot of treatment once all the disease had been diagnosed.

In comparison my experience in private practice exposed me to patients who predominantly came in with aesthetic concerns and had fairly healthy if not completely healthy mouths. The appointment times were longer, and the dentists seemed to have more time to spend with the patient.

The ability to help so many patients and provide so much care to those who would not be able to fully afford it on a completely privatised system highlighted a huge benefit of working on the NHS. However seeing some treatments available privately to patients who are maintaining their oral health but have other concerns causing them emotional or psychological distress I feel I would like to have the option to be able to offer these patients' treatment options as well. Therefore in my opinion a career which incorporated both NHS and private work would work best for me."

NOTES

Chapter 10

OTHER GENERAL QUESTIONS-
DESIGNED TO MAKE YOU
THINK OUTSIDE THE BOX

1.Have there really been any dramatic changes to the NHS since it was founded?

2. What is wrong with the NHS?

3. What does the World Health Organisation do?

4. What is the difference between NHS and private dentistry?

5.How do you think the dental profession has changed over the last 25 years?

6.What is the biggest challenge facing dentistry today?

7.What is the future of dentistry?

1.Have there really been any dramatic changes to the NHS since it was founded?

The NHS has not really changed in its principles since it was founded in 1948. Care is still free at point of use, except for prescriptions and dental charges, everyone is eligible for care (even visitors to the UK), and it is funded by government collected taxes. It is still based on the system of the GP being the "gatekeeper" to hospital services, and hospitals being run by regional organisations

What has changed is the way in which the system is run. Originally run as a giant organisation, it was with the 1990 NHS and Community Care Act, that a culture of an internal market was formed. This meant that local authorities and some GPs would be able to act as buyers of services from hospitals and other organisations, in the hope that this would increase competition and raise standards. The new Health and Social Care bill passed in 2012 is the greatest threat to the fundamental structure of the NHS. By abolishing the regional organisations which run hospitals, and giving more power to GPs to buy services from hospitals, it makes hospitals more vulnerable to competition and could lead the way for a more privatised healthcare system.

Read more about the short history of the NHS at
www.nhshistory.net

*"I think that the values of the NHS remain the same
as it always has been , which is to provide free
healthcare to all paid for by taxpayers. In recent
times, the emphasis on patient satisfaction has been
pushed to the forefront, which I believe is important,
however the new healthcare reforms put in place are
the most dramatic changes to the NHS. It abolishes
the regional healthcare authorities responsible for
the hospitals and replaces them with GP run
organisations. This move presents the greatest
change in NHS culture as local health authorities
were established with the founding of the NHS, but
also it now means GPs are more responsible for the
financial burden of healthcare, which poses its own
ethical dilemmas."*

2. What is wrong with the NHS?

You could be talking about it all day if asked this question. However what is currently wrong with the NHS is that there is not enough money in the system. What is the reason? As most clinicians will tell you, it is because it's almost impossible to count the cost of illness. One patient's pneumonia could take 3 weeks to clear, while another just one. This results in an extra 2 weeks which cannot be price-coded in the same way. Similarly another person's appendectomy could take an hour long than the next resulting in having to pay staff one more hours wage in order to complete the operation. Across the NHS, inability to account for the unexpected nature of illness means that attempts to treat all patients equally and fairly undermines the values of running a cost effective service. However despite this, there are ways to save money while making services efficient enough to deal with patients, and this is what the NHS needs to focus on. Cutting unnecessary management costs in order to re-organise and reshape its services to where they are needed the most.

If you choose to focus on a particular area of the NHS, ensure you know a bit about the problem in order to be prepared if discussed in more detail.

"The NHS has many problems, and as an outsider, I couldn't really make a judgement on what is wrong with the NHS itself, however I believe that the nature of its business, in dealing with unexpected illness leaves itself vulnerable to the costing of illness, as there is no way to be able to budget for procedures and treatments for different patients, as they could react totally different. Its not the same as a consumer based system, where the customer asks for what they want and they get it and are happy. The NHS deals in making people well, and as long as the treatment is covered by NHS guidelines, it means that for as long as it takes, treatment will be given until deemed not in the patients best interest, and this could cost much more than expected. I think this is one of the reasons that the NHS have a big financial problem."

3. What does the World Health Organisation do?

The World Health Organisation (WHO), is a specialist department of the United Nations which deals with international public health. Founded in 1948, it was charged with improving public health across the globe to allow people to attain the highest possible level of health, particularly in the fields of communicable and sexually transmitted diseases as well to improve maternal and child health.

Its major triumph as a organisation has been its leading role in the eradication of small pox, while currently it leads the way in fighting HIV/AIDS around the world as part of the UNAIDS network. The two other major communicable diseases which it aims to combat is malaria and tuberculosis.

Learn more about the WHO and some of its success stories which you can talk about if ever asked from the WHO website. www.who.int

"I know that the World Health Organisation is an UN organisation responsible for international public health. It produces the World Health Report which is a leading publication on health and is also organises the World Health Day. I know that it produces many reports on the health status of various diseases as well as working to reduce the effect of communicable

diseases on populations around the world. Recently work on reducing congenital rubella syndrome in children by introducing measles and rubella vaccines in initiatives around the developing world has been extremely successful, with WHO plans to eliminate measles and rubella in more than 80% of the world by 2020."

4. What is the difference between NHS and private dentistry?

NHS dentistry has a central focus on clinical practice. This includes all of the dental treatments necessary to achieve and maintain good oral health care. This may also include treatments that help to restore the function of dental health in the most cost- effective way possible. This means that treatments that are aesthetic in nature (ones concerned with improving one's appearance, such as cosmetic dentistry procedures) are not included in the list of treatments provided by the NHS.

Private Dentistry on the other hand focuses on the clinical aspect alongside the aesthetic need of a patient. The prevention and treatment of dental problems entwined with improving a patient's smile is what private dentistry is all about. When thinking of costs; Private dentistry prices are not fixed (unlike those under the NHS), therefore, the cost of dental treatments under private dentistry dentists tend to vary a lot, depending on the location of the practice, the technology to be used, the complexity of the treatments, and the individual case's needs.

"Dental care provided by the NHS is delivered on the same principle as healthcare- high standard of care, accessible by all! However this accessibility is only for patients with dire clinical need to help keep their mouth, teeth and gums healthy and free of disease. During my work placement I learnt that treatments like dentures, crowns, bridges, can be provided by the NHS dental care. In addition, dental implants and orthodontic treatment like braces can also be covered as long as there is a medical need to justify it. Private dentistry on the other hand is run by dental practitioners themselves and provides a combination of clinical and aesthetic treatments at a range of different prices. The dentist I shadowed explained to me that this variation is based upon a combination of factors, from the location of the practice, the technology that is used in the treatment, the complexity of the actual treatment and the individual patient's needs."

5.How do you think the dental profession has changed over the last 25 years?

"Dentistry is an ever changing profession with advances in techniques, materials and technologies. The ethos leaning towards being preventative of disease and minimally invasive. Amalgam had been the material of choice for many years, but with material advancement, composite (white fillings) have been developed to be used in situations (e.g. very deep cavity) where amalgam was the material of choice. The NHS contract introduced in 2006 (and currently still in place) is unit of dental activity based, and was an attempt to improve and monitor access to dentists. The contract, currently being piloted, to come into effect in 2014 is based more on prevention rather than activity of treatments.

6.What is the biggest challenge facing dentistry today?

We are on the cusp of a change in contract in the coming year or so (2014). The challenge faced will be the adaptation to the new systems and ensuring a smooth changeover occurs so as not to affect patients. Along with this dental phobia is amongst one of the most common phobias in the UK. With the new preventive health orientated contract it is hoped the patients don not perceive the dentist as simple 'drilling and filling'.

7.What is the future of dentistry?

This question wants to know what you know about dentistry and from what you know where do you think its going. Read some news on dentistry and look on websites like dentistry.co.uk or ukdental news.co.uk to be up to date with current affairs and ongoing news.

"Even though oral health has improved in the past few decades, there is still a significant amount of dental disease to prevent and treat. Prevention is a lifelong commitment with regular checkups. It is hoped the future of dentistry will be preventative and health driven. It is hoped this will have a more positive impact than the current situation."

Chapter 11

OTHER GENERAL QUESTIONS-DESIGNED TO MAKE YOU THINK OUTSIDE THE BOX

1.If you were the head of a group of dentists and a colleague was not doing the job well what would you do?

2. If you were asked to design four stamps to mark the 50th anniversary of the NHS what would you put on the stamps and why?

3.If you where the prime minister what three government policies would you set to achieve?

4. Give me examples of the roles that dental nurses play in the modern healthcare system?

5. Give me your opinion on how do you think the health system should be funded?

6. European Working Directive - what do you know about them?

7. Who are the General Dental Council?

8. Where do you see the health service going in your opinion?

9. What do you know about the British Dental

Associations?

10. Describe this image (any image/painting could be shown to you)

NOTES

1.If you were the head of a group of dentists and a colleague was not doing the job well what would you do?

Think about how you would respond to a team member that was not pulling their weight. Although there is technically no right answer, they are looking to see that you will be able to deal with people in a team environment in an appropriate manner.

Remember that giving a team member the opportunity to improve by first offering feedback is the often the first line of helping to improve performance within a team.

"As the head of the group, I would look to understand why my colleague was not doing their job appropriately. This would involve a personal consultation with the team member finding out if they had any particular problems and offer support if they did. I would also highlight any deficiencies which I would suggest they could improve on. We could then review things after a time period in order to monitor how things were progressing. If there were no improvements, this would result in thinking about more serious implications for the involved parties if needed."

2. If you were asked to design four stamps to mark the 50th anniversary of the NHS what would you put on the stamps and why?

"The stamp designs which I would choose would be:

The iconis blue and white NHS logo – this is because it is an instantly recognisable logo associated with all things healthcare in this country. Every building, vehicle, and paraphernalia linked to the NHS is branded with the logo, and could work well if presented in a different colour to the regular blue and white.

A picture of doctors and nurses at work – as these professions are the backbone of the NHS it would make sense to show them at work in a hospital environment.

A portrait picture of Aneurin Bevan – He was the health minister in 1948 who unveiled the dream of bringing good healthcare to all financed by central taxation. As the "founding father" of the NHS it would be appropriate to honour him though a postage stamp.

A picture of some backroom staff such as porters, cleaners and administrators – to highlight that the NHS needs all these people in order for it to run as effective as it does. "

3.If you where the prime minister what three government policies would you set to achieve?

Think of sensible achievable policies which are currently being employed and think of ways in which you could improve them. This can be a much detailed answer if need be, however think of trying to summarise the key points of the policies which you would focus on.

"As prime minister I would focus on government policies which would improve healthcare but through less direct means.

I focus on healthcare organisation and efficient running of NHS hospitals in order to reduce deficits

I would improve provision for social care in order to make sure that there was enough resources to look after the elderly particularly those who are more vulnerable in order to reduce bed-blocking.

Finally I would invest in public health initiatives such as increasing exercise and eating more healthily to continue to improve the general health of the nation. Problems such as obesity, diabetes and hypertension are preventable and is key to reducing cost of treatments."

4. Give me examples of the roles that dental nurses play in the modern healthcare system?

In the modern healthcare system, the role of the nurse has been extended for a number of reasons. Demand on the remit of the dentist means that more responsibility shared with other healthcare professionals means more efficient use of time, while more educated and engaged nurses allowed for better care for the patients.

Nurses within a dental practice carry out the following duties amongst others:

They adhere to cross-infection and health and safety protocols to the highest standard.

They ensure that all the required equipment is adequately disinfected after every single patient and dental instruments are decontaminated appropriately.

They set up the correct instruments, prepare the room and get the notes ready for each patient coming to see the dentist

They perform the role of an assistant to the dentist during treatment by passing relevant instruments and equipment, aspirating and retracting when necessary.

They monitor the patient from the moment that they

enter the treatment room, all the while during treatment and as they leave the surgery.

They offer support and reassurance to patients and also carry out stock control

Being able to spend time with dental nurses during your work experience would be an invaluable time spent as they can carry out many tasks alongside dentists on a regular basis.

5. Give me your opinion on how do you think the health system should be funded?

As an opinion question you are entitled to say whatever you feel as long as you can justify why you have said it. There is no right or wrong answer as explained previously. However have a good structure to your answer as always, think about what the problem currently is, what you are suggesting, why you are suggesting and how it could be achieved.

"I believe that currently the funding of the health system is inadequate and taken advantage of by individuals as they feel that it is their right to expect treatment regardless of cost despite their contribution to taxpaying. Although it is a good principle, I think the NHS should be semi-privatised, so that each person is given a certain budget and if

172

their treatments exceed this, they will have to pay the remainder. This would reduce the amount of people who abuse the health service with minor ailments, but also mean that care would be improved as more money would be available for improving the semi-privatised services."

6. European Working Directive - what do you know about them?

The European Working Time Directive is a law passed by the European Union which must be followed by its member states, of which the United Kingdom is one. It entitles each worker to have

a minimum of 20 days of leave in a full time job

a daily rest of 11 hours in a 24 hour period

no more than 48 hours working in a 7 day period.

This has had huge implications on the shift patterns on doctors as it means that on-call shifts have effectively been shortened to no longer than 12 hours. However in the UK it is possible to opt out of the 48 hour week rule and work longer hours. Some may see it as a step forward in protecting patients from tired, over-worked doctors, but many clinicians have felt that it often means that junior doctors lack the experience of being in hospital which helps them become better doctors.

"I know that the European Working Time Directive is a EU law which has changed the working patterns of doctors, particularly junior doctors in the UK, restricting them to 48 hour weeks and no longer than 12 hour days. Although this makes for less tired and stressed doctors, it also has any implication on staffing and the level of exposure for junior doctors as they are in hospital much less than before."

7. Who are the General Dental Council?

The GDC are an organisation which regulates dental professionals in the United Kingdom. This includes all dentists, dental nurses, dental technicians, clinical dental technicians, dental hygienists, dental therapists and orthodontic therapists. All the above stated must be registered with the General Dental Council in order to work in the UK.

They set the standards of dental code practice and conduct and ensure that professionals keep up to date, whilst working to strengthen patient protection.

8. Where do you see the health service going in your opinion?

With the new NHS healthcare bill being approved recently, the NHS could go in a number of directions. One which has particularly concerned many observers is the fact that more power going to GP consortia and increasing internal competition means a shift to towards patients having to pay for certain services which could eventually lead to a fully privatised healthcare service. Feel free to express your opinion if they asked, as long as it's reasonable.

"I think that with the introduction of the new Healthcare Bill which see greater power going to GPs in the form of consortia and a greater emphasis on internal competition, this leads the NHS open to new challenges. The main one would be preventing new private competitors from taking patients away from NHS hospitals, thus, weakening the health system, and eventually leading to the rise of private hospitals. This could lead to a semi-privatised system, whereby patients would have to pay for certain services, and in the long term, to a fully privatised insurance based health system similar to the US."

9. What do you know about the British Dental Associations?

The British Dental Association is a professional association and trade union for dentists in the United Kingdom and was founded in 1880. As this is an organization that is not owned by any external members, it functions solely for advancing science, arts , ethics and general dental practice for its members. Once you buy membership you gain a lot of support and advice on the NHS rules and regulations, other governing bodies, meet and liaise with other colleagues at national/international BDA meetings. Furthermore, there is ample guidance on dental literature, medline searches and they also provide guidance on employment law and health and safety in practice. (Read more at www.bda.ord)

10.Describe this image. Why have we asked you to do this?

The image could be of absolutely anything so this is not about second guessing what the image could be of. They may even ask you to describe this to a blind person (or pretend you are describing this to a blind person). This question wants to see how well you can articulate what you can see, how understandable what you articulate is for a blind person to create the image in their head. It also tests your ability of assessing something and describing the big general picture first BEFORE you dive into any fine details about anything. The key here is to NOT TUNNEL VISION straight into any finer details before explaining what the bigger picture is about. This avoids you missing anything out!

Having answered this question the examiner may ask you why they asked you to describe a picture. There are a few reasons;

Dentists know their profession in fine detail and this may not be understandable to their average patient so they need a way of conveying this information to the patient. Appropriate articulation enables the patient to make an informed choice on their treatment.

Dentists have to analyse images on a regular basis (e.g. radiographs). To correctly identify any evidence of disease and convey this onwards a dentist needs to have a systematic approach to assessing.

Communication skills are important in being able to describe things well to another person, for example another team member etc.

"This is a landscape A3 sized painting of what looks like a country side house, by a lake, with a boat in it on a sunny afternoon. In the backdrop there are some green hills top left and the sun in a clear sky on the top right. The brick house is on some land to the

177

left of the centre of the image, with the white boat in the middle of the lake. [Then describe individual parts in detail]

When asked why you can use the answers above."

Chapter 12

CURRENT AFFAIRS BASED QUESTIONS

1. Do you read newspapers? Name an interesting dental related story.

2. How do you go about keeping up to date with current dental issues?

3. What do you read of a dental nature?

4. Tell us about any medical/dental articles you have seen in the media recently?

5. What do you believe has been the biggest breakthrough in dentistry?

6. What was the last book/article you read about dentistry?

7. What major issues are currently affecting the NHS?

8. How do you think dentists are viewed in the current media?

9. What do you consider to be important advances in medicine over the last 50 years?
10. How do you think the rise in technology has influenced and will continue to influence

the   practice   of   dentistry?
11. What do you think are the downfalls of health informatics and increased provision of technology?

12.If you did not get onto the dentistry course, what other profession would you be interested in?

13. What makes a good team member?

1. Do you read newspapers? Name an interesting dental related story.

Reading daily or weekly newspapers is important for your own personal development in making sure that you are up to date with current issues as well as taking in well written opinions about what is going on in the world. Any publications however are good enough, and with the emergence of tablet pcs, often publications are accessible in a paperless form. Make sure you have read through a number of current magazines or newspapers which you can talk about at your interview if asked a question such as this. Always try to reflect on the piece and critically analyse it using your own judgement in order to show that you have insight into a particular topic.

Here are some key things that you need to try and memorise so that when you talk about the article/paper that you read, it all sounds very credible and articulate.

WHEN ?

The year that it was published

" I recently read a paper in the BDJ which was published earlier this year..."

"I recently read a very interesting article on the BBC website which was published almost a decade ago... and I was surprise how aspects of it still rung true

181

today..."

WHO?

The author (this will look really impressive)

" I recently read a paper in the BDJ which was published earlier this year, written by Professor XYZ..."

"I recently read a very interesting article on the BBC website which was published almost a decade ago, written by Mr 123, a renowned journalist ... and I was surprised how aspects of it still rung true today..."

WHAT?

A brief summary of the article

"the cohort size was 250, which is quite big and hence I felt that the results could have some significance.... "

WHY?

Your view on what the author's ulterior motive was in writing the piece

"although this was written by a dentist himself, he could have had alterior motive of promoting his own practice in comparison to others....

"I usually like to read the Daily Telegraph as well as The Times as my regular newspapers. One article in the Telegraph which caught my eye of recent was an article scrutinising dentists for putting patients at the risk of infection by not cleaning their equipment properly. I found this really interesting as during my work placement the dentist was meticulously thorough with his sterilisation technique. The report claims one in 9 dentists inspected by the Healthcare watchdog were guilty of these shortcuts, but it made me think about where those dentists were, in terms of location, demographic and what time of day were they inspected as this finding didn't ring true of the practices which I volunteered with. This was an article which was published early last year and it would be really interesting to see if this trend continues in the years to come"

2. How do you go about keeping up to date with current dental issues?

This question is asking how do you show your interest in the field of dentistry through reading, and it is important to show that you do so via a variety of reliable methods. Always be prepared to talk about a current article you may have seen from the sources you mentioned.

Newspapers although good for reading, lack concrete scientific grounding, often paraphrasing from real science to fit their purpose.

Magazines such as New Scientist are well rounded scientific publications which help broaden your knowledge of science around the world.

The internet is the main source of information in the world today, many websites have health sections such as the BBC, where you can search for numerous scientific journals and abstracts in the fields which you are interested in.

"I usually keep up to date with current dental issues via a number of ways. I try to keep up daily by visiting a website called dentistrytoday.com which collates sources from a variety of journals such as the BDJ as well as other news sources to deliver dental news, it is usually the first place I go to read about developments in , while I also use the BBC Health website to look at more British focused news articles. Furthermore I subscribe to the New Scientist magazine, which I find to be a really good read, updating me on current medical, dental and scientific news while having a range of interesting articles."

3. What do you read of a dental nature?

Reading more specific journals and dental magazines highlights a more direct interest in the field of dentistry, journals like the student British medical Journal, for example are great entry level journals for young people to read.

"I like to read the student British Medical Journal which has a range of interesting articles, including tips while being in medical/dental school and ways to improve studying and learning. As well as this it keeps me up to date with developments in the medical world both in the UK and abroad. I thoroughly enjoy the way that it is written and hope to continue to subscribe to it if I get into dental school."

4. Tell us about any medical articles you have seen in the media recently?

Like mentioned before, always be prepared to talk about a few medical/dental articles which have recently been in the news, as they will be expecting you to know about the biggest stories. As usual reflect on the news article and put it into society context.

"One interesting article, I read on the BBC News health website recently talked about the risks of moderate drinking on the dementia risk. A longitudinal study in the US was found to showed that women in their 60s who drank a moderate amount of alcohol, around 7-14 units of alcohol increased their risk of developing problems with memory and brain functioning. They also found that fortnightly binges also increase the risk of dementia like symptoms in both men and women. TI believe that if the research has some truth, this could have huge implications on future generations of Britons given our "binge drinking" culture and the massive rise in women drinking much higher quantities of alcohol."

Note: it is unlikely that you will be asked this question, but once again it is included for a well rounded depth

5. What do you believe has been the biggest breakthrough in dentistry?

There are hundreds of new advances in dentistry happening each year, by keeping abreast of the latest dental news, you will be able to talk about one which has interested you enough to believe that it has been the biggest. This is another opinion question and so as long as you can justify why you think it's the biggest then the answer will be A*.

"I believe one of the biggest breakthroughs in dentistry has to be the cosmetic affair of teeth whitening. Not only has it shifted from once being a luxurious treatment to a cosmetic 'must-have', but the use of materials and procedures such as peroxide whitening, laser whitening and even home whitening kits have made that perfect smile accessible to all."

6. What was the last book/article that you read about dentistry?

Reading dentistry related books, may be slightly premature as you may not have a place in dental school, but be positive and don't be afraid to see what dentists are reading in order to align your mind frame early. Reading books which may give you an insight into the dental career are definitely more useful at this stage of your education to help you make a more informed decision about medicine.

"The last dental related book I read was a book by David Clow 'A few words from the Chair'. It was a book which I found at a family friend's house and which I thought may be an interesting read in allowing me to understand more about the patient's perspective and concerns in the experience of visiting the dentist. It gave me insight on the barriers to

effective dental care- the primary one being patient anxiety. I found this really interesting as I had never thought about that aspect of delivery of care before this book "

7. What major issues are currently affecting the NHS?

The NHS are affected by a number of issues, and the news agencies in the UK do not fail to highlight them, with almost a news article a day commenting on the NHS. Keep abreast with any current scandals or long running problems by reading more topical news articles and websites such as the BBC Health website.

"I know that currently the major issue facing the NHS is its financial management, particularly in this time of austerity. In the news recently there has been articles relating to the massive debts faced by the South London Healthcare Trust which puts 5 major South London hospitals in danger of closing some departments or even whole sites. It is due to be put into administration which is a worrying prospect as there must be hundreds of thousands of people who rely on those hospitals, and if any were to close, it would have a significant impact on the entire region."

8. What do you consider to be important advances in medicine over the last 50 years?

"I believe that one of the most important advances in medicine over the last 50 years has to be the completion of the Human Genome Project which has opened a new chapter in the treatment of not only genetic diseases but also of conditions such as diabetes and hypertension which have certain predisposing genes which can now be identified in order for us to study its cause more carefully. It has revolutionised the way that we diagnose, treat and manage patients with genetically linked diseases as well allowed the medical world to create simple and effective screening tools to prevent certain diseases manifesting. I think that better knowledge of our genome is also vital to help us develop better treatments which can be used for even more diseases which we dong quite understand, and think that this is one advance which will continue to help the field of medicine grow."

9. How do you think the rise in technology has influenced and will continue to influence the practice of dentistry?

Technological advances go hand in hand with medical/dental advances and are needed in order for dentists to be able to test the boundaries of practice in a safe and secure manner. Technology allows information to be processed quicker than we as humans can manage, as well as being the backbone for newer more efficient imaging techniques, diagnostic tools and results reporting. The switch from paper to electronic records is also vital in making sure patient care can be monitored more closely and information shared amongst healthcare teams much quicker. Give some examples of the technological success stories which are driving dentistry.

"I think that the rise in technology is the most important factor in influencing how medicine and dentistry is now practised in the developed world. The advancement of computers mean that better imaging techniques such as MRI and CT can be used there are always new programs being developed for these, while it also allows more and more information to be processed electronically, such as patient records, results and managing patient treatment plans. Even in surgery, robots allow surgeons to be more precise in the operations which they do, reducing human unsteadiness and error. The internet also allows the instant transfer of information both for learning and treating patients meaning that doctors around the world are more informed about medicine in general. I believe that this will continue to drive the medical field in the future and that nearly all of the medicine which doctors practise will require some sort of

technology."

10. What do you think are the downfalls of health informatics and increased provision of technology?

An increase in the provision for technology is the answer for the future, but think of some of its limitations. Increasing the delivery of advanced technology may result in the doctor's role being marginalised (e.g. in Telehealth where consultations can happen over the computer) but in dentistry this same increased provision empowers the dentist. As a dentist's predominant role involves his hands, and top of the mark equipment, any advances in technology will only add to the proficiency and effectiveness of the consultation. The only other downfall may be the problems in implementation of any new software, as it takes time and money to both train and equip the staff to become ready to use the software.

11.If you did not get onto the dentistry course, what other profession would you be interested in?

Dentistry is one of the most competitive courses to do at university and receives one of the highest number plications. There is more chance of you not ing into dental school than succeeding so you ast be prepared for the what you would do if your application this year is unsuccessful at whatever stage. Although you may have wanted to do dentistry all your life, try to use a question like this to re-evaluate your life. Think about the skills you have and how you could apply them or excelled in other professions. You could do this with the background of re-affirming your desire to do dentistry!

"If I didn't get onto the dentistry course, I would definitely want to try again as I believe that dentistry is the career path which I want to take, and would use another year to improve myself and my application to ensure I got in on second time of asking. I don't have an alternative career choice at the moment, but I think that I would make a good mathematician as I have a very logical mind and Maths is one of my favourite subjects at AS level."

12. What makes a good team member?

Teamwork is essential in the healthcare setting and being a good team member is vital for ensuring the team operates at its highest level possible.

Attributes of a good team member:

Not complacent

Does not exert their own ego

An effective communicator

Willing to listen to others opinion

Able to give and receive constructive criticism

Contributes to team discussion and effort

Works hard to ensure the goals of the team are met

Puts the needs of their team above personal desires

These are just some of a few attributes of which a good team member is seen to have, with the most important being that you are willing to be cooperative with your team's efforts regardless of relationships within the team. In your answer feel free to highlight examples of when you feel you have been a good team member or some of the things which you do to help be a better team member in the teams you are a part of.

"I believe that being a good team member is essential in the healthcare profession and in all walks of life where a group of people are needed to achieve a common goal. As part of my school football team, I have had the experience of seeing what helps make a good team player, with many of our team being great examples, which has been part of the reason for our recent cup successes. I think that a good team member works hard for the team regardless of their position, is able to share in the responsibility of the

team, both in its success and failure, and is able to communicate well in order to make sure everyone around them knows what's going on. I know that my experience of being a part of my school football team has allowed me to understand what a good team player is and I hope that it will stand me in good stead for the future."

<u>Notes</u>

Notes

Notes

Notes

Found this book useful?

Consolidate everything you have learnt by attending the dental interview course and one-to-one tutorials by medinterview

Book now

-www.medinterview.com-

Use the code VBitloml397 for £50 discount that comes with the purchase of this book.

Made in the USA
Monee, IL
16 April 2020